WRITING IN PSYCHOANALYSIS

WRITING IN PSYCHOANALYSIS

Francesco Barale *Parthenope Bion Talamo*
John E. Gedo *Patrick Mahony*
Henning Paikin *Fausto Petrella*
Giorgio Sacerdoti *Antonio Alberto Semi*

CRC Press
Taylor & Francis Group
Boca Raton London New York

CRC Press is an imprint of the
Taylor & Francis Group, an **informa** business

First published 1996 by Analytic Press, Inc.

Published 2018 by CRC Press
Taylor & Francis Group
6000 Broken Sound Parkway NW, Suite 300
Boca Raton, FL 33487-2742

CRC Press is an imprint of Taylor & Francis Group, an Informa business

ISBN 13: 978-0-88163-239-2 (hbk)
ISBN 13: 978-1-138-87229-5 (pbk)

Visit the Taylor & Francis Web site at
http://www.taylorandfrancis.com

and the CRC Press Web site at
http://www.crcpress.com

CONTENTS

INTRODUCTION

This is the first volume of a monograph series, *Psychoanalytic Issues*, published jointly by the *Rivista di Psicoanalisi* (journal of the Italian Psychoanalytic Society) and Karnac Books. The series, and in particular this first volume, is primarily the result of deliberations within the editorial board, initiated when Alberto Semi became Editor-in-Chief three years ago. In addition, it addresses a long-standing problem—the relative isolation of our Psychoanalytic Society as a result of language barriers. It is true that such is the fate of most psychoanalytic communities that do not use English as their main language—their scientific debates are seldom communicated to other linguistic groupings. And we may all agree that it is a terrible waste to develop ideas if they cannot circulate freely and be open to confirmation and refinement.

We believe that there is a great contrast between the liveliness of much scientific discourse in our midst and communication abroad. The international scientific literature is widely read in Italy, both in the original and in translation. Consequently, our members are keenly aware of developments on the international scene; this diffusion of information is largely responsible for the pluralism that characterizes our psychoanalytic community. We feel it is incumbent upon us, at this point, to overcome the failure to communicate with our colleagues abroad—to master our partial aphasia, so to speak. Hence it is no coincidence that we initiate our monographic series in English with an issue devoted to "writing in psychoanalysis".

All this might sound as though we had had some grand general plan in mind when we decided to initiate the series. Actually, we were at first unable to avail ourselves of anything so sophisticated, the whole project having grown in a more elementary manner, somewhat evocative of the growth of organic matter—by "accretion", as it were. The *Shorter O.E.D.* defines this process variously as "Continued growth. . . . The growing together of particles, or of parts normally separate. . . . The process of growth by external addition . . .", and so on.

The nucleus of this particular volume saw the light following a November 1993 colloquium organized by Semi for those involved in publishing the *Rivista*. The aim of this meeting was to discuss the many problems involved in writing and, consequently, the particular difficulties of editorial work. The idea was to reflect both on the intrapsychic and the relational dimensions at stake: in particular, concerning the latter, we felt that, as psychoanalysts involved in editorial work, an elaboration of the relationship between us and the authors who sent their papers in for evaluation was crucial. The meeting was extremely stimulating, and the papers were published in Issue 4, 1993, of the *Rivista*, as a way of communicating to the readers of the journal not only the meaning of our work as editors, but also the meaning that their work had for us, over and above the technicalities involved in the evaluation of a manuscript. We thought it might be interesting to hear what analysts from other psychoanalytic cultures, also engaged in editing a psychoanalytic journal, might have to say on the subject, and, since responses were encouraging, it was decided that it might be worth while publishing our efforts, having further expanded the process of growth by the addition of contributions by colleagues from other psychoanalytic cultures.

We are grateful to John Gedo, Patrick Mahony, and Henning Paikin not only for the intrinsic value of their respective papers, but, above all, for their readiness to contribute to this volume, thus sustaining our belief in the vitality of a truly common psychoanalytic culture, transcending the limits imposed by differing idioms. To this end, the theme of the present monograph appears to us a particularly apt one. After all, the history of writing in psychoanalysis is part and parcel of the history of the psychoanalytic movement—from Freud onwards, all psychoanalysts have felt the need to write psychoanalysis and have wrestled with the difficulties involved.

The Editors

WRITING IN PSYCHOANALYSIS

CHAPTER ONE

The reveries of a solitary scribbler

John E. Gedo

I suspect it is the sheer volume of my psychoanalytic publications that elicited the invitation to contribute an essay to this symposium. I was fortunate enough to earn my psychoanalytic qualifications at a relatively early age, so that I have had almost four full decades of opportunity to practise the craft of writing in psychoanalysis. My career could well be characterized by the mocking *bon mot* once used to deprecate Edward Gibbon, "still scribbling. . . ." How many pages have I published? (How many trees have I caused to be destroyed?) I have not kept count, but I suspect that, among living colleagues, none is guilty of greater volubility. It is not for me to claim that my output has been weighty, but it certainly occupies more than my fair share of shelf-space. Consequently, I feel justified to approach our topic from a very personal vantage point.

Nothing angers me more than overhearing detractors who dismiss my contributions because, according to them, I "know how to write". (The implication is that this skill is an illegitimate trick through which hollow ideas are made to seem solid.) Not that I am alone in suffering such attacks: the American analyst whose work I most respect, Robert Gardner (see Gardner, 1983,

1984, 1995), is frequently put in his place by his writings being called "poetry". I read them as cogent essays in epistemology, stated with the clarity and economy sadly lacking in most psychoanalytic texts. W. B. Yeats has reminded us that one cannot separate the dancer from the dance—neither can the writer's concepts be separated from the form in which they are communicated. Over 90 years ago, Freud rightly asserted that good writing is the consequence of clear thinking about one's subject matter (Freud, 1901b, p. 101). Nobody is born with a talent for scientific discourse.

On apprenticeship

By now, almost everyone knows the New York story about the lost *Ausländer* who asks an old peddler how to get to Carnegie Hall. "Son", the wise man replies, "practice! practice! practice!" Writing is no different from playing the violin (or basketball)—the skill must be acquired by practice. The youthful Balzac threw away the manuscripts of more than half a dozen novels before he broke into print—some two thousand pages of mere rehearsal; the psychoanalytic writer can scarcely hope to master his craft with greater ease.

In this regard, the education of most psychoanalysts—by no means only those who enter the field from medicine or psychiatry—tends to be deficient, for it seldom involves much serious challenge to produce written work that is to undergo stringent criticism by qualified judges. I have also been extremely fortunate in receiving opportunities of this challenging kind: in secondary school, by successively having to master communicating in three different languages (as my family moved in stages from Central Europe to North America); in my undergraduate years, by being offered rigorous courses in English composition, British and French literature, and more history than hard science; and even in medical school, where I was permitted to spend much of my last year writing for a students' yearbook and creating a play satirizing the faculty. It was Freud's *panache* as an expositor that attracted me to psychoanalysis, and I never doubted that joining the profession would permit me to continue writing.

When young people interested in becoming *littérateurs* ask for advice about how best to achieve this ambition, they are usually told that they should read as much good literature as they can. (Of course, it is not sufficient to read for content alone: *Macbeth* is not a murder mystery, nor is any of Freud's case histories merely a narration intended to highlight an individual's personal drama.) I have the impression that would-be psychoanalytic authors all too often neglect to follow worthy literary models. (Is this neglect of attentive reading particularly prevalent in North America, where television threatens to push the printed word into obsolescence? Perhaps so—but, *Heute Los Angeles, Morgen die ganze Welt*[1]. . . .) At any rate, my future as a prolific writer of psychoanalysis was prefigured when I matriculated at the Chicago Institute and found that I was inclined to read more psychoanalysis than anyone I encountered. For decades, I read most of the principal journals (in English) from cover to cover, as soon as they appeared. I did not find most of this material particularly valuable *qua* contributions to psychoanalysis, but thinking through why this was so, particularly in terms of the way the papers were organized, was enormously instructive.

The value of these exercises was soon validated by my experience as a reader of manuscripts submitted for publication to various journals, particularly the *Journal of the American Psychoanalytic Association* and *The Annual of Psychoanalysis*. These publications use at least three readers to evaluate every manuscript and ask them to submit detailed reports that specify the reasons for their recommendations. These reports and the Editor's letter to the author about the disposition of the submission are then shared with each reader. I believe this is an excellent method for checking the reliability of the referees. I have now participated in well over a hundred evaluations performed in this manner and was gratified to discover that in the vast majority of instances the readers were in unanimous agreement. (I tend to reject more papers than my fellow referees, mostly because I value originality, in addition to the essential virtues expected by everyone. I can remember only one paper I endorsed because of its conceptual novelty that was ultimately turned down; others thought it was overly speculative.) At any rate, with practice I have gradually learned to evaluate psychoanalytic writings more and more expeditiously: nowadays, I find it possible to write reviews of most analytic books after a single reading, without bothering to take notes.

I mention this gain in efficiency because I believe it shows that with sufficient study of the writings of others, one may master the proper organization of psychoanalytic publications. Needless to say, writing a book is a more complex enterprise than is the production of an essay, so that a would-be author of monographs had best prepare by writing careful book reviews. Before I became a regular contributor to the analytic literature, I managed to get myself appointed as Book Review Editor of the *Journal of the American Psychoanalytic Association*; for about five years, I regularly wrote brief reviews of some 10 volumes annually for this journal. Needless to say, to keep up this pace it was imperative to grasp the author's intention and methods quickly and to assess the adequacy of the book's structure as well as the validity of its argument. I have also learned a great deal from writing formal surveys of the entire analytic literature about certain topics (see Gedo, 1970, 1972) and from systematic reviews of the life work of certain analytic authors (see Gedo, 1968; 1973; 1981, ch. 11; 1986, ch. 3–8). I cannot claim that I have succeeded in avoiding all the pitfalls I thought my predecessors had fallen into, but I have certainly tried to do so. In summary, there are no short-cuts to writing psychoanalysis *comme il faut*: it requires hard work and adequate preparation.

On quality

Of course, one may train oneself to write adequately and still produce only trivia: in this regard, writing in psychoanalysis does not differ from writing in general. Many are called, but few are chosen. In my judgement, at least half of the published analytic literature is devoid of merit. On the basis of my editorial work for a number of journals, I am also convinced that our publications do not overlook worthy manuscripts—on the contrary, they tend to compromise their declared standards in order to fill their allotment of space. All over the world, psychoanalytic journals and publishing houses proliferate faster than do the scholarly/scientific capabilities of our discipline. The inevitable result is the printing of blather.

Among the numerous causes for the publication of well-written trivia, the one I would pinpoint as most prevalent is the failure of many authors to familiarize themselves with previous contributions on their subject. Of course, with the geometric expansion of our written production, the task of adequately surveying the literature has become ever harder. We have probably reached the point of needing a computerized data base to accomplish this important job thoroughly. A few psychoanalytic libraries (again, fortunately for me, including the one at the Chicago Institute) have computerized their own holdings, but none of them owns a complete set of the whole corpus of psychoanalysis, particularly of the materials published in languages other than its own. If psychoanalysis aspires to reach a literary standard comparable to that of other scholarly fields—from accounting to zoology—we must urgently establish a world-wide computer network linking all of our libraries.

It should also be stated explicitly that the failure to take into account significant prior work often results not from the difficulty of finding these references, but from a cavalier dismissal of the value of contributions by adherents of schools of thought different from the author's. The tendency to cite only those publications that stem from one's own intellectual circle has been one of the most important intermediate steps leading to the fragmentation of psychoanalysis into factions that do not communicate with each other. In recent years, I have even noted a trend to ignore ideological opponents deliberately, as a political manoeuvre to smother their potential influence. If my impression is valid, this development is an alarming departure from the psychoanalytic (and scientific) ideal to search for Truth and humbly to submit one's efforts to reach it for reasoned comparison with those of others. Of course, it has always been difficult to live up to these ideals; perhaps because of the current fashion to cast doubt on the very concept of Truth, they seem no longer to be shared by all of us. If every conviction were really determined by narcissistic considerations, as deconstructionists imply, how would psychoanalytic discourse differ from a political campaign?

At the same time, it must be admitted that various traditions within psychoanalysis have had such a long history of autochthonous development that it is scarcely feasible to correlate their respective positions on any particular issue with each other. Even if this lamentable state of affairs has not quite supervened as yet, the effort to compare one's thesis to those of contributors from an alien tradition may be more trouble than it is worth. As one example among many one could mention, let me recall a Franco–American psychoanalytic *Rencontre* in Paris, about a dozen years ago: the French audience was utterly bewildered by a paper by an adherent of ego psychology; the American participants were scandalized by the cavalier manner in which most French presenters attempted to support their contentions. My own presentation (Gedo, 1981, ch. 10), a clinical thesis based on developmental considerations, was perceived by an intelligent French discussant as a tyrannical effort to put a theoretical strait-jacket on the analyst's free exercise of some function I did not understand. *Mamma mia!*

At any rate, it is always a difficult balancing act to give proper consideration to the relevant literature without going too far afield. *Cogent* writings in psychoanalysis must show an awareness of the current conceptual structure of our entire intellectual domain—a standard ever more difficult to meet as a result of the centrifugal forces fracturing the field. Even if we lower our expectations and demand only thorough mastery of the author's specific psychoanalytic tradition, most of our publications fall short of seeing the sub-field in question whole. As a result, much of our literature is busy reinventing the wheel, claiming originality for pouring old wine into new bottles, and oversimplifying human behaviour by espousing some fashionable *pars pro toto*[2] fallacy. Of course, we should let every flower bloom, despite the sad fact that most plants in our garden are weeds.

On necessity and solitude

Most psychoanalysts never publish at all or, at best, write only an occasional paper; the list of *writers* in our ranks is surprisingly limited. (Of course, in this regard, psychoanalysis is no different from any of the other "health professions": battling disease is not conducive to the *vita contemplativa*.) Our failure, thus far, to find a secure place as an academic discipline within the established university system has deprived all but a handful of exceptions among us of the opportunity to devote our professional life to scholarship. As private practitioners, we are obliged to subsidize our own scholarly activities, and most of us lack the resources to do this without impairing our standard of living. (Needless to say, the potential market for serious psychoanalytic writings is too restricted to make such scholarly work profitable.) I cannot say that I have been impoverished because I devoted fewer hours to remunerative work than my colleagues, but I *have* been chagrined by the stigmata of their greater prosperity, and I attempted to redress the balance by demanding higher fees than most. These are unavoidable complications, and they doubtless deflect many potential contributors from the path of writing psychoanalysis.

Even more discouraging is the solitude necessary for the task of the writer—a lack of actual human contact that psychoanalysts (whose choice of profession betrays a strong preference for dyadic relationships) may find particularly opprobrious. (For more detailed discussion of my view on the psychological vicissitudes that affect creativity, see Gedo, 1983, 1996.) To put this another way, to write psychoanalysis, one must obtain the cooperation of one's entire family. (As Anna Freud once told me, both she and her mother "devoted their lives" to make it possible for her father to produce his oeuvre.) I know several gifted colleagues who have been unwilling to extract such sacrifices from reluctant family members. To echo Yeats once again, they opted for perfection in life over perfection in work. I have never been confronted with such a painful choice, for my wife has been immersed in scholarly activities for almost as long as myself (see M. Gedo, 1980, 1985, 1987, 1988, 1994).

All in all, to write psychoanalysis requires vaulting over so many hurdles that it is scarcely an exaggeration to say that this track will only be followed with perseverance by that small group of colleagues who by writing respond to an inner necessity. (In this regard, it is well to remember that there has long existed a great tradition of medical authorship, from Galen through Maimonides and Rabelais, to Anton Chekhov, Conan Doyle, Freud, Jung, William Carlos Williams, Lewis Thomas, Oliver Sacks, and countless others. And it is possible to emulate these great predecessors simply by writing psychoanalysis. . . .) I have the impression that the most productive authors in the psychoanalytic domain have been "writers first"—individuals who stumbled into the clinical arena more or less against the grain. Take a figure such as James Strachey, whose *magnum opus* was the *Standard Edition* in English of the entire Freudian oeuvre: this analyst was a member in good standing of the Bloomsbury group, related to such eminent *littérateurs* as Lytton Strachey, who, in turn, revolutionized the art of biography by infusing it with psychological insight. Or take Ernest Jones, whose massive *Life of Freud* and sparkling autobiography have outlasted his other works (Jones, 1953, 1957, 1959).

On genre and method

At various stages of my psychoanalytic development, I have been drawn to writing projects of very different kinds, in large part because I knew that they called upon those skills, abilities, and experiences that I had at my disposal at the time. Today, I would be utterly unable (and decidedly unwilling) to engage in the painstaking preliminary research required to produce the work on the intellectual history of psychoanalysis that was my stock-in-trade as a psychoanalytic author during the early years of my writing career. (I collected most of these papers in a volume co-edited by Pollock—Gedo & Pollock, 1976, ch. 1, 3–5, 7–8, 11–12, 15.) Those labours are best performed by persons with more energy and ambition than I am now able to command—not to speak of the physical demands of long hours of attentive reading, note-taking, searching for references, and so on. I am now better equipped to write spontaneous reveries while I sit in my swivel-chair and look out on the distant horizon over the waters of our inland sea. But it has taken a lifetime of steady publishing to embolden me to follow wherever my pen might lead me, in the conviction that editors and readers will be satisfied with the result. Of late, I have not hesitated to present myself as a psychoanalytic Jeremiah—or Cassandra (see Gedo, 1984, ch. 10–12, 14; 1991, ch. 12–13). In emulation of Rossini's *Sins of my Old Age*, I am even planning to write a set of *Memoirs*, full of spleen. (Perhaps that project will no longer constitute "writing in psychoanalysis", but it is the most challenging assignment I have ever given myself as an author, because its success will depend entirely on its literary qualities.)

It is not surprising that one is best qualified to write about psychoanalytic problems about which one has pondered for years, even decades. Rushing one's *premières pensées* into print seldom yields fruitful results; allowing them slowly to marinate has the additional advantage of permitting one to determine the proper focus on the issue and to digest at leisure whatever other contributors might have to say on the subject. I often find that, when I want to start writing about some topic, I am overcome by a conviction that I am unready to tackle it. I have learned never to disregard such a message from the depths. It generally does not cause me to abandon my plans, but I now always wait until I feel certain that I have a clear thesis and I know how to present it. It is only then that it pays me to start writing. A blank sheet in a typewriter has never elicited a paper from a would-be author who is unprepared, and the purchase of a personal computer is not likely to solve this *contretemps* magically.

In my own case, I have become convinced that a sense of being ready to write about a topic means that I have preconsciously organized whatever I can say about it so that, when I begin the actual composition, I can rely on producing a coherent manuscript without first making explicit to myself what I intend to present. In other words, I focus exclusively on creating the sentence I need to express a given idea; when that sentence is complete, I invariably find that the next idea necessary for my exposition will automatically present itself. (Of course, in preparing a first draft, I do not concern myself with details of punctuation, word order, or finding *le mot juste*. Matters of that kind can gradually be taken care of while I revise the manuscript and—if it is accepted for publication—at the stage of copy-editing or checking the printer's proofs.) I know that working in this manner would not suit everyone, but for me it has been an extremely efficient method; much of the time, my initial drafts of individual essays require little or no revision. Obviously, giving a monograph the best organization possible is a more difficult challenge, and I have reshuffled the manuscripts of my books more than once. [This was the case with my first two books (Gedo & Goldberg, 1973; Gedo, 1979) as well as my most recent (Gedo, 1996). In contrast, a book based on a set of lectures informally delivered as a visiting scholar in Jerusalem (Gedo, 1988) required little revision.] On occasion, the critiques of editors or friendly colleagues have suggested solutions for problems of organization I had been unable to overcome on my own.

Over the years, I have dabbled in every genre of psychoanalytic writing, and I have found some of them much more congenial than others. I suspect that my experience is fairly typical: most of us find it maximally challenging to write a meaningful, reliable, and convincing case history. As an author, I take greatest pride in having published extensive psychoanalytic case histories in greater numbers than anyone else, sometimes at considerable length. (The most detailed are contained in Gedo, 1979, ch. 4, 6, 8; 1984, ch. 4, 5; Gedo & Gehrie, 1993, ch. 2.) It is very difficult to provide sufficient observational detail to allow the reader to follow one's reasoning in reaching one's interpretations, without prolixity or—even worse!—lapses into irrelevance. It is all too easy to present unsubstantiated inferences in lieu of clinical data—particularly because we lack consensus about what *has* been substantiated in psychoanalysis. (Thus the case reports of our ideological opponents always read like a string of arbitrary assertions without empirical referents—a potpourri of fictive entities.) It is best to omit the construct language of psychoanalysis from case reports, but describing the course of a psychoanalytic encounter in the plain vernacular takes narrative skill of a high order. It is particularly difficult to present such material in a condensed form: the more detail we eliminate, the more crucial choices must be made about what constitutes the heart of the story. Freud's case histories were sometimes attacked because they had the impact of novellas—of course, it is precisely their formal excellence that has earned them classical status. Alas, the writing of short stories is an art supremely difficult to master.

In my experience, the only genre that presents a comparable challenge is work in the interdisciplinary arena. In order to produce something of relevance to both disciplines involved, not only must the author learn up-to-date bodies of information in each; what is even more daunting, the unique epistemic methods of psychoanalysis have to be made to mesh smoothly with those appropriate for the other field concerned. Failure to address this methodological problem has defeated most efforts in this domain. Inevitably, good results often require consultation with experts in the other discipline or even explicit collaboration with them (see Baron & Pletsch, 1985, ch. 3–10, 16; Moraitis & Pollock, 1987, ch. 18). I have sometimes ventured into exercises in psychoanalytic biography (mostly in the service of exploring creativity—see Gedo, 1983, 1996; Gedo & Gedo, 1992), but I have seldom dared to tackle subjects clearly within the boundaries of the humanities or social sciences. I must confess, however, that I have fantasies of spending my retirement writing psychoanalytically about the operas of Mozart . . .

Envoi

Psychoanalysts often behave as if the expansion of our discipline were equivalent to progress. In my judgement, this illusion is equivalent to the belief that one has automatically made a profit by selling commodities after a bout of inflation. The steady growth of our membership has inevitably (and justly) brought demands for democratization in its wake; the triumph of such egalitarian ideals has made it difficult to make unfavourable qualitative judgements about the writings of our peers. As a consequence, the over-all standards of our current literature are considerably below those prevalent when I entered the field in the 1950s. Obviously, I agree with my fellow Chicagoan, Mies van der Rohe, that often "Less is more".

NOTES

1. *Heute Los Angeles, Morgen die ganze Welt:* Today Los Angeles, tomorrow the whole world.
2. *Pars pro toto:* a part for the whole.

CHAPTER TWO

Psychoanalysis—the writing cure

Patrick Mahony

According to a medieval maxim, anyone who claimed to have read the whole corpus of St. Augustine would most probably be a liar, since the writings of that great thinker were so voluminous. I believe that a similar maxim might hold true today for Freud, if we were to have also at our disposal the stupefying quantity of both his destroyed manuscripts and his extant but still unpublished writings. But there is another pertinent reason that I have started my presentation with Augustine. He made two incisive comments about what writing can mean to an indefatigable author, and Freud could just as well have said them about himself. The first comment, coming from Book Three of the Latin treatise *De Trinitate*, can be rendered this way: "I myself avow that in writing (this work) I have learned many things which I did not know" [*"Ego proinde fateor me ex eorum numero esse conari, qui proficiendo scribunt et scribendo proficiunt"*—Augustine, *Omnia Opera*, 2: 690]. The second, more poignant citation comes from Letter 143, which I

From: *Cahiers Psychiatriques Genevois*, Special Issue (1994): 101–119. Reprinted by permission.

translate as follows: "Admittedly, therefore, I try to be among the number of those who write as they progress and who progress as they write" [*"Egoque ipse multa quae nesciebam scribendo me didicisse confitear"*—Augustine, *Omnia Opera*, 8: 1218].

We might use one more medieval reference in order to see how writing was crucial in Freud's own development. Scholastic philosophers were wont to distinguish between an *instrumentum separatum* or instrument detached from the user (such as a hammer) and an *instrumentum coniunctum* or instrument connected with the user (such as his hand). In light of this distinction, we may say that Freud's writing was carried out more or less like an extension of himself, a tracing of his inner movement. For another enlightening gloss, we may turn to Roland Barthes, perhaps the foremost Continental critic in our day on the subject of writing. Barthes distinguished between a writer, for whom writing is merely a communicative instrument, and an author, who establishes the very way of discourse and "who radically absorbs the world's *why* in a *how to write*" (Barthes, 1964, p. 148; my translation). In this sense, Freud is clearly an author—a genuine, committed author who experienced writing as a mixture of work and pleasure. He would have sympathized with Barthes, who reflected on his own prolific activity this way:

> Writing is that *play* by which I turn around as well as I can in a narrow space: I am boxed in. I struggle between the hysteria necessary to write and the imaginative act, which oversees, guides, purifies, renders common, codifies, corrects, and imposes the aim (and vision) of a social communication. . . . And yet: the closer I get to the work, the deeper I go into writing; I approach its unendurable depth: a desert is discovered. . . . It is at this point of contact between writing and work that the harsh truth appears to me: I *am no longer a child*. Or rather, is it the asceticism of intense pleasure that I am discovering? [Barthes, 1975, p. 140; my translation]

The latter quotation leads us directly into the most tortuous and exalted portion of Freud's writing career called his self-analysis. Freud conducted it through, with, and in writing. Far from being a mere medium of retrospective reportage or a way of storing and retrieving information, writing was an indispensable feature with the deepest significance in Freud's self-cure. Such is my thesis, and in the course of pursuing it, I wish to elucidate the origins of psychoanalysis, the quality of Freud's genius, and the distinctiveness of that world masterpiece, *The Interpretation of Dreams* (Freud, 1900a).

Before moving on, we must attend to several preliminary questions. First of all, when did Freud's self-analysis take place? In our reply, we must start by dividing his self-therapy into two stages: a kind of initial, non-systematic one that began around the time that Freud was treating the patients that we can recognize in the *Studies on Hysteria* (1895d); then an intensified, systematic self-analysis that began in the summer of 1897 and, with interruptions, lasted at least up to the publication of the *Interpretation of Dreams* in November 1899 (see Appendix). I do not want to burden the reader with dates, but it is important to retain the dates more or less marking the duration of Freud's systematic self-analysis: from the summer of 1897 to November 1899.

It is not a trivial gesture to ask what material Freud's self-analysis focused on. Documentation amply shows that parapraxes, symptoms, and screen memories were worked on in his self-analysis, yet its principal material—and not at all incidentally—revolved around dreams. Again and again, Freud himself was very explicit on this matter. In 1909 he told his American audience at Clark University: "If I am asked how one can become a psychoanalyst, I reply: 'By studying one's own dreams'"! (Freud, 1910a, p. 33). Three years later, Freud returned to his historical pronouncement and repeated it word for word in a paper on technique (Freud, 1912e, p. 116). Next, in his history of the psychoanalytic movement, Freud reminisced this way about its earliest days:

> I soon saw the necessity of carrying out a self-analysis, and this I did with the help of a series of my own dreams which led me back through all the events of my childhood: and I am still of the opinion today that this kind of analysis may suffice for one who is a good dreamer and not too abnormal. [Freud, 1914d, p. 20]

Finally, in 1926, endorsing a paper by a certain English thinker, Freud wrote that its author "carried out a systematic application of the procedure of self-analysis which I myself employed in the past for my own dreams" (Freud, 1926c, p. 280; cf. Jones, 1953, pp. 320–321; Gay, 1988, p. 98 fn.).

The next problem confronting us, the practical modality of Freud's self-analysis, leads us further into the unique history of psychoanalysis. It is a historical irony that a name frequently used for psychoanalytic treatment, the talking cure, had been coined for a very different kind of therapy and one, moreover, that preceded Freud's discovery of psychoanalysis by more than a decade.

The story is familiar: Anna O, Breuer's patient from 1880 to 1882, would jokingly refer to her cathartic treatment as "chimney-sweeping" but in a serious mood would call it a "talking cure" (Freud, 1895d, p. 30). A second ironical disparity of psychoanalytic history is that the other source of our clinical practice, Freud's self-analysis, was preeminently not a talking cure (nor merely a reflective, non-motoric one, for that matter) but a writing cure. (For a while, however, it seems that Freud did analyse himself silently and without recourse to writing—Freud, 1895d, pp. 284, 294.) The evidence for my thesis—both circumstantial and direct—is extensive.

First, concerning the circumstantial evidence, it is relevant that in citing the historical precedents for free association, Freud drew attention to the fact that they had transpired in writing. For example, Freud noted that the nineteenth-century scientist Dr. Garth Wilkinson had described his own manner of writing as an enraptured laissez-faire, letting himself be guided "by an infallible instinct into the subject" and its elaboration. Another predecessor, now much better known, is the essayist Ludwig Börne, who said that to become an original writer one had only to engage in sheer scriptory improvisation for three days. We know the cryptomnesic history of this essay: the young Freud read it, but then for over half a century it slipped deep into an unconscious transcription in Freud's own mind (Freud, 1920b, pp. 263–265). An even more telling precedent is one brought up in the *Interpretation of Dreams* itself: Schiller, let us recall, held that free association on paper is the way to overcome writer's block. Freud himself added this practical comment:

> What Schiller describes as a relaxation of the watch upon the gates of Reason, the adoption of an attitude of uncritical self-

> observation, is by no means difficult. Most of my patients achieve it after their first instruction. I myself can do so very completely, *by the help of writing down my ideas as they occur to me.* [Freud, 1900a, p. 103; italics added]

The documentation that I have thus far adduced prompts us to conceive that Freud's self-analysis was chiefly a written one dealing with dreams. But there are much more pertinent data for our conception. A generally neglected footnote in the *Studies on Hysteria* shows that as far back as the time of its composition Freud took the trouble with some of his fresh dreams "to write them down and try to solve them" (Freud, 1895d, p. 69 fn.). Freud's writing practice assumed even a greater role at the climactic point of his non-systematic self-analysis. Although it was in the course of analysing the Irma dream that Freud discovered the secret of dreams, critics have overlooked how that dream and its immediate history are literally bathed in writing: being uneasy about his therapeutic treatment of Irma and wanting to lay the blame elsewhere as well as justify himself before Breuer, Freud sat down late in the day and wrote up the patient's case; the write-up was not done cursorily, for it lasted "far into the night" (Freud, 1900a, p. 108; cf. also pp. 106, 115). According to Freud, this case history, plus some alarming news about Irma's condition, continued to occupy his mental activity after he fell asleep; he then had the famous dream about her. Pertinent to my thesis, the most condensed part of the dream was a chemical formula, which Freud even visualized in bold type. Immediately upon waking, on the morning of 24 July 1895, Freud noted down the dream; he then analysed it, part by part. The dream, therefore, whose most dense section was in print, was itself bracketed by two phases of writing—in other words, day residues and associations were in written form. That is not all. On the same day that Freud analysed the dream, he wrote to Fliess, but he did not mention the writing-up of his epoch-making discovery. Like his dream, Freud's letter was accusatory and—given the topic of my presentation—its opening words become even more charged: "Demon, why don't you write? . . . Don't you care at all any more about what I am doing" (Freud, 1895d, p. 134).

The foregoing information enables us to become more attuned to the scriptory modality of Freud's systematic self-analysis that began two years after the Irma dream. During this later period, Freud hyperin·ested in the inscription of his dreams and associations and his analysis of them—a praxis that expanded to include his screen memories, parapraxes, transient symptoms, and interactions with patients. It is quite to the point that also at around this time Freud saw an uncanny resemblance between his compositional practice and that of an inspired Biblical writer; hence, while scorning the arbitrary devaluations made by his predecessors, Freud claimed that he was closely attending to dreams, as if they were "Holy Writ" (Freud, 1900a, p. 514). What is more, in recording his own dreams, the practice of free association drove Freud to act like an inspired writer. Accordingly, in reporting his so-called Hollturn dream, Freud declared:

> This description is unintelligible even to myself, but I am following the fundamental rule of rendering the dream in those words which occur to me in writing it down. [my translation of G.W. 2/3, 458 ff.; see Freud, 1900a, p. 455 fn.; cf. also pp. 205, 456]

Barely a few months after completing *The Interpretation of Dreams*, Freud set forth in the most direct terms his precise method of self-analysis and improvised writing:

> If we make use of this procedure [of free association] upon ourselves, we can best assist the investigation by *at once* writing down what are at first unintelligible associations. [Freud, 1901a, p. 636; emphasis added]

Freud thereupon proceeded to jot down and analyse, in the present tense, the dream he had had the night before. (See the German text in the *Gesammelte Werke*, 2/3: 649 ff., which renders the dream and its associations in the present tense. The resultant immediacy contrasts with the effect of distance brought about by Strachey's recourse to the past tense—Freud, 1901a, pp. 636 ff.)

The scrupulous method Freud adopted to analyse his dreams, we may say, actually involved him in more rather than less writing. As he said at one point, the "original, classical method" of analysing one's dreams was to skip nothing: in practice, it meant chopping the dream into sequential parts and then dutifully proceeding to associate "to the elements of the dream in the order in which those elements occurred" in the dream report (Freud, 1923c [1922], p. 109). Clearly, this methodical pursuit of the dream from its start to its end eliminated the risk of any random procedure that would easily have resulted in overlooking some dream segments. Another writing strategy of Freud's is more intriguing and relates subtly to his general clinical technique. Freud said:

> If the first (dream) account given me by a patient of a dream is too hard to follow I ask him to repeat it. In doing so he rarely uses the same words. But the parts of the dream which he describes in different terms are by that fact revealed to me as the weak spot in the dream's disguise. [Freud, 1900a, p. 515]

We do, in fact, have a few of Freud's own dreams with slightly different written versions, a discrepancy due either to a defensive reaction or to a conscious desire to disguise his dream in published form. But in other instances, such as the dreams that lend themselves to diagrammatic presentation, it seems that Freud tended to rewrite them for the purpose of discovering more through his own associatively spatial rearrangements. For example, in presenting his well-known succinct dream about closing the eyes, Freud states: "I am accustomed [*gewöhnlich*] to write this in the following (diagrammatic) form" (Freud, 1900a, pp. 317–318; G.W. 2/3: 322–323). We must take the word "accustomed" for exactly what it means—not just two or three times, but many times. The implication is clear: Freud wrote the dream down a number of times to find out the meanings hidden in the various ways he could graphically display it. For another example, we may refer to the Villa Secerno dream, which Freud sent to Fliess with the comment: "*The way I have written it out* shows what seemed obscure and what seemed multiple" (Freud, 1895d, p. 236; italics added). Significantly enough, Freud wrote out this dream differently in *The Interpretation of Dreams* (1900a, p. 317). [Of the four journals on dreckology or anality that Freud wrote, at least three contained dreams—Freud, 1985d, pp. 291–301. Although Freud was avowedly writing the journals for Fliess (p. 301), he had not sent the first one, which contained "wild dreams" that were, Freud said, "part of my self-analysis" (p. 291). Such a declaration makes it clear that Fliess was not privy to all of Freud's self-analysis.]

We can hardly exaggerate the importance of the fact that Freud retained his writing method in his self-analysis even when he dealt with material other than dreams as such. Here Freud is reporting a flash memory about his early childhood:

> I saw myself standing in front of a cupboard demanding something and screaming, while my half-brother, my senior by twenty years, held it open. Then suddenly my mother, looking beautiful and slim, walked into the room, as if she had come in from the street. These were the words in which I described [*gefasst*] the scene, of which I had a plastic picture, but I did not know what more I could make of it. Whether my brother wanted to open or shut the cupboard—in my first translation [*Übersetzung*] of the picture I called it a "wardrobe"—why I was crying, and what the arrival of my mother had to do with it—all this was obscure to me. [Freud, 1901b, p. 50; G.W. 4: 59]

Note Freud's technique: much as he did with dreams, he wrote down the screen memory and closely heeded the original wording, which he called a "translation".

Inscription, transcription, translation—these terms were frequently used by Freud to describe the so-called psychic systems and the vicissitudes of their traces; the triad of terms casts light on what writing both as a concept and as a practice signified for Freud. In a practical sense, the place of writing in his self-analysis was partly determined by his innate gifts as well as by external circumstances. Thus, for a considerable period during his writing cure Freud forsook giving his university lectures (Freud, 1895d pp. 332, 347). Even more significantly, throughout his writing cure, Freud did not achieve any talking cure with his patients. [The most influential of these patients was Mr. E; we know specifically of two dreams by Freud about this patient (Freud, 1900a, pp. 435–439, 455–459). Through dreams and memories about his nanny and his childhood libidinal attraction to "*matrem nudam*" (Freud, 1985d, p. 268), Freud discovered his own Oedipus complex and was "on the way to grasping its universal application"; thus, Freud's belief in oedipal universality was confirmed, not initiated, by one of Mr. E's dreams (Freud, 1901b, p. 178—for a chronologically reversed and erroneous interpretation of this influence, see Anzieu, 1975, p. 331).]

Throughout Freud's letter's to Fliess (Freud, 1895d), one can see a chronological series of his epistolary laments:

- in March 1897: "I have not yet finished a single case" (p. 232);
- later in the same month: "I am still having the same difficulties and have not finished a single case" (p. 233);
- in May 1897: "I shall wait still longer for a treatment to be completed. It must be possible" (p. 244);
- in September 1897: "[I have] continual disappointment in my efforts to bring a single analysis to a real conclusion" (p. 264; cf. p. 269);
- in February 1898: "I shall not finish a single one [case] this year either" (p. 299).

Even as late as March 1900, we hear Freud bemoaning the elusiveness of the case which he most counted on to resolve his doubts and to have confidence in his dyadic therapy (Freud, 1895d, p. 403). To gauge the bleakness of Freud's therapeutic mood further, in the same letter in 1898 in which he said that he would not finish a case in that year either, Freud announced that he had just finished composing *Sexual Aetiology of the Neuroses*, an essay that contained the following propagandistic and misleading claim: "I have in recent years almost worked out a therapeutic procedure which I propose to describe as *psychoanalytic*. I owe a great number of successes to it" (Freud, 1898a, p. 282). In short, such contrasting contemporary private and public statements about the success of the talking cure certainly point to Freud's personal embroilment, and it is reasonable to conclude that his preeminently written cure took on that much more importance.

At this juncture one may want to object that Fliess played a major role in Freud's analysis (cf. Gay, 1988; Jones, 1955, pp. 6, 387, 482; Freud, 1895d, p. 73), and that although they were in contact with each other through the post, they did also communicate with each other verbally during their so-named Congresses. To that objection, I would answer that we must not overestimate the extent of those dyadic encounters. We are sure that there were at least five of them during Freud's systematic self-analysis, but there may have been one or two more.[1] Yet several points must be borne in mind here. The Congresses usually lasted for only one or two days. Next, there was something about these Congresses that conformed to the ordinarily accepted sense of the word, for both men tended to deliver papers to the other or to read silently what the other had written (see, specifically, Freud, 1985d, pp. 287, 335, 344, 349). Thirdly and most importantly, available evidence suggests that the Congresses were essentially intellectual exchanges.

For these and other reasons, therefore, we must not underestimate the role that writing played in Freud's relationship with Fliess. From the outset of their acquaintanceship, Freud envisaged successful writing as a shared ego ideal. In Freud's very first letter, to his appeal for friendship is added a report of compositional production: he is busy writing three essays (Freud, 1985d, p. 16). In his second letter, Freud states his intention to translate a book and adds that "for recreation" he is working on two papers (Freud, 1985d, p. 17).

But, by 1897, Freud's disenchantment with his friend started to surface, for published research, successfully written up and published, came more and more to be a hypersensitive issue between the two correspondents. [The poetic activity of Freud's son, Martin, began in April, 1897 (Freud, 1985d, p. 236) and, through a strange historical fate (identification with his father) seemed by October 1899 to be petering out (p. 377).] We must realize here that Freud's disillusionment concerned not only Fliess's theoretical stance but also his lack of production as such; and in this matter Freud did not have in mind merely a comparison of his own psychological achievements with Fliess's biological work. Indeed, it has generally gone unnoticed that between 1887 and 1900, the years when their friendship was relatively positive, even Freud's neurological publications alone far exceeded in length Fliess's biological ones. To be more specific: between 1887 and 1900 Fliess published two monographs and, from what I can determine, four short articles, the whole totalling fewer than 400 pages. Just to mention Freud's neurological books for the same period, we have, in addition to the book on aphasia, a monograph written with Oscar Rie and containing some 220 pages and a bibliography of 180 titles; then a 168-page monograph dealing with central diplegias; and, lastly, a comprehensive treatise of some 327 pages and 14 pages of bibliography (Jones, 1953, pp. 216–217). Let us not forget either that along with reading and summarizing the massive extant literature on dreams, between 1898 and 1900 Freud published 83 abstracts and reviews of neurological literature (in the *Jahresbericht über die Leistungen und Fortschritte auf dem Gebiete der Neurologie und Psychiatrie).* If, finally, we also take into consideration, for the overall period between 1887 and 1900, Freud's numerous articles on his own neurological research, the mass of his psychological publications, and his translations of three books by Bernheim and Charcot, we begin to grasp the breathtaking unmatchability of Freud's creative powers and productivity.

In this whole scenario, 1897 was the watershed year for our two protagonists—Freud finished his last book on neurology (in January), and Fliess saw a book that he had completed the previous year appear in print (Freud, 1985d, p. 173). Between 1897 and 1900, however, Fliess wrote nothing but one short article. It is no surprise that reality-testing became a burning issue in the famous friendship, as Freud resorted to an impatient pressuring so that Fliess would come forth with documented evidence of successful work. A chronological sampling of excerpts in Freud's correspondence shows dramatically his growing impatience with Fliess's scriptive unproductivity:

> June, 1897: "(I hope) that instead of a short article you will within a year present to us a small book which solves the organic secrets." [Freud, 1985d, p. 254; cf. p. 304]
>
> February, 1899: "You can write of nothing but the tremendously huge work which is all too hard for the powers of a human being." [ibid., p. 314—in this same letter Freud said that he himself had just discovered the key between dreams and neuroses]
>
> May, 1899: "A contented letter from you containing evidence of your being well and the promise that you will attempt a first presentation of your earthshaking formulas were a long-missed pleasure." [ibid., p. 351]
>
> June, 1899: "The announcement that you are engaged in research perhaps may mean, (that) instead of writing? And

(thus the) postponement of the date on which I can read something of yours?" [ibid., p. 356]

August, 1899: "Your work apparently has changed into a pupa for me: will I be able to catch it as a butterfly, or will it fly too high for me?" [ibid., pp. 365–366]

If we reflect on these passages and others, we can draw the assured inference that Fliess's promise of his own great book to keep pace with the *Interpretation of Dreams* was becoming more desperate. [At the beginning of 1900, however, there was a two-month lull in Freud's writing (Freud, 1985d, p. 404).]

The supreme irony was that Fliess was caught on the tenterhooks of his own theory about life's periodicity: he could not predict when he would finish that very book of his that Freud wryly called the "organically growing creation" (Freud, 1985d, p. 428). As a matter of fact, the work did not see the light of day until many years later, in 1906.

The preceding discussion prepares us to examine the composition of the *Interpretation of Dreams*, which is a fascinating story in itself. We begin in 1908, when Freud prefaced the second edition of his dream book with the following information: "It was, I found, a portion of my own self-analysis, my own reaction to my father's death—that is to say, to the most important event, the most poignant loss, of a man's life" (Freud, 1900a, p. xxvi). Freud's retrospection needs some filling in and modification. His father died in October 1896: in May of the following year, Freud began writing the dream book (Freud, 1985d, p. 243) but quickly ran into a self-described writer's block (pp. 253 and 255). Psychoanalytic scholars have overlooked that this very writing block launched Freud into the systematic self-analysis which eventually culminated in his resumption of writing the *Interpretation of Dreams*. This compositional feature, embracing a unique mixture of scientific and therapeutic goals,[2] was such that only after the completion of his masterpiece did Freud realize that the very writing of it formed part of his self-analysis. [Earlier during his self-analysis Freud considered the writing of his book to be an alternative activity (Freud, 1985d, p. 299). But by the middle of 1899 he postulated an analogous relationship between the two activities—cf. the highly significant expression, "as it were" (Freud, 1900a, p. 477; G.W. 2/3: 481).] In his letter of 16 May

1897, Freud gives a historical announcement about undertaking the dream book. His inaugural wording of that project is of the utmost importance: "I have felt impelled to start working on the dream, where I feel so very certain" (Freud, 1985d, p. 243).

Freud hyperinvested in the dream material, for it was precisely there that he felt most certain. Also, Freud's feeling of being "impelled" [*gedrängt*] is one of his recurrent references to his manner of inscriptive work at the time: again and again he speaks of having taken notes during the last "thrust" or waiting patiently for the next "thrust" (Freud, 1985d, e.g., pp. 243–244, 249, 300, 301, 349). Another point about Freud's inaugurating announcement is that he uses the word "dream" to refer to his whole project. In the German text of his correspondence with Fliess, we repeatedly hear Freud talking of his writing project as the "dream" [*Traum*]; the English translation editorially adds the word "book" in brackets, thus detracting from the force of Freud's condensation of dream book into "dream". The accumulated force and impact of Freud's condensation is undeniable. By the end of 1897, he is saying: "I shall force myself to write the dream in order to come out of it" (Freud, 1985d, p. 278). "The dream is suddenly taking shape . . . the dream will be", Freud would later say (p. 353). And later again: "[I am] entirely the dream" (Freud, 1985d, p. 369; German edition, p. 403; my translation).

Freud's verbal condensation was more than a figure of speech. Family members noticed that when he was composing his monumental treatise, he was in a dream-like state (Jones, 1953, p. 360 fn.). And even he himself wrote to Fliess: "The psychology is proceeding in a strange manner; it is nearly finished, composed as if in a dream" (Freud, 1985d, p. 318). This process of writing the dream book is telling, for the processive nature of Freud's understanding process is inseparable from his written presentation. Here is Freud again, confiding to Fliess:

> I can compose the details only in the process of writing. [Freud, 1985d, p. 305; cf. p. 146]

> It is entirely taken down [from the dictation] of the unconscious. . . . At the start of every paragraph I did not know where I would end up. [ibid., p. 319; German edition, pp. 348–349; my translation]

> I do not know yet how to delineate and organize (the last chapter) . . . but a thing like this turns out just as it will. Every attempt to make it better by itself gives it a forced quality (ibid., p. 368).

The foregoing evidence entitles us to conclude that Freud's discourse in most of his dream book is truly performative and ongoing. Its quintessential character is epitomized by the usage of the present tense, and in that way it has the grammatical nature of the manifest dream. Accordingly, more than being just the result and account of Freud's self-analysis, the *Interpretation of Dreams* enacts and extends it. [Compare the somewhat disparate statements in Anzieu, 1975, pp. 590 and 661. This shaky conceptualization extends to Anzieu's other position that when there is a coincidence of two or three of the dream book's directive personages (dreamer, interpreter, narrator, theoretician), Freud becomes paralysed. But at least the first three coincide in Freud's enactive prose.]

Put in another way: at the time dreaming and writing were not so much collateral as imbricated activities for Freud—an imbrication that could even become collusive. Did not Freud write to his friend, "So far I have always known where the next dream-night would continue" (Freud, 1985d, p. 268)? And when Fliess insisted that a certain important dream be dropped from the monograph, Freud yielded but went on to ask which of the dream's particular elements Fliess objected to—the reference to anxiety, to Martha, or to being without a fatherland? Whatever the objectionable elements, Freud added, he would eliminate them in one of his future dreams, for he could "have dreams like that made to order" (Freud, 1985d, p. 315). It follows, then, that Freud's book about dreams was also a dream to a certain extent. Dreams and book cartwheeled in a series of mutual wishes and fulfilment. The dreams were texts and pre-texts.

Were we to stop at this point, we would not fully grasp the extent to which Freud was more personally involved in writing *The Interpretation of Dreams* than any other book. Our exploration of this personal involvement leads us to see that, in Freud's mind, there was a profound link between dreams and the maternal body.

Here are excerpts from two strategic places in *The Interpretation of Dreams* (ch. 2 and 7):

> Every dream has at least one place . . . a navel, as it were, by which it joins with the unknown. [Freud, 1900a, pp. 116 ff.; G.W. 2/3: 116 ff., my translation]

> Then this is the dream's navel, the place at which it straddles the unknown. [Freud, 1900a, p. 525; G.W. 2/3: 530, my translation]

These two lapidary expressions anticipate another: "The finding of an object is the refinding of an object" (Freud, 1905d, p. 222). In his dream the dreamer re-finds, "joins with", and even "straddles" the mother, the unknown. (Strachey's desexualized rendering of *aufsitzt* or *straddles* is "reaches down into" (cf. Freud, 1900a, p. 525; Weber, 1982, p. 75.)

The suggestive power of Freud's statements is increased by the fact that the word in German comes from a verb [*erkennen*, not *bekennen*] (Anzieu, 1975, p. 215), which, like the English *know*, can be used in the biblical carnal sense. Let it be stressed that the two appearances of the word "unknown" function as mileposts marking the exploratory distance travelled by Freud in his dream book. In the first citation, drawn from chapter 2, the dream's navel is merely joined with the mother; this controlled attachment is matched by the main material of chapter 2, the Irma dream, whose deeper meanings about the maternal body were given a restricted interpretation by Freud. However, towards the end of his exploration of the dream, in chapter 7, Freud could speak allusively about the dreamer straddling his mother. Such a libidinalization of Freud's writing is brought closer to home when we attend to the larger elements of discursive strategy in the dream book.

The dream book combines both exposition and narrative: if the focus of its exposition, the dream, is symbolic, so are the scene and movement of its narrative. In the clearest terms Freud explained the investigation in his book as a journey through nature—both its landscape, symbolic of the female genitalia, and woods, generally symbolic of the mother (Freud, 1900a, pp. 355, 684; 1916–1917, pp. 156, 159–160). Freud wrote privately to Fliess:

> The whole thing is planned on the model of an imaginary walk. At the beginning the dark forest of authors (who do not see the trees), hopelessly lost on wrong tracks. Then a con-

> cealed pass through which I lead the reader . . . and then suddenly the high ground and the view and the question: which way do you wish to go now? [Freud, 1985d, p. 365]

If in this letter the dark forest designates the dream book's introductory historical survey of oneiric literature that was first urged by Fliess (Freud, 1985d, pp. 354–355, 362), in another letter Freud indulges in a more suggestive description: the introductory chapter is a thorny brush wood [*Dorngestrüpp*] in which most readers will get stuck; they may never proceed beyond it to see the Sleeping Beauty [*Dornröschen*, literally, little thorny rose or hedge rose] (Freud, 1985d, p. 362; G.W., p. 397). As we know from the Grimms' fairy tale to which Freud is referring, Sleeping Beauty—or the embodiment of perfect femininity—struck by the curse of an evil fairy, is finally revived through the kiss of a rescuing prince. In Freud's private imagination, of course, both he and his ideal reader would be such daring co-conquistadorial princes.

Also, in the *Interpretation of Dreams* Freud imagistically maps out his investigation as a journeying through a maternal landscape. The exposition in chapter 2 is symbolically identified as "passing through a narrow defile" (Freud, 1900a, p. 122); at this point, Freud says that a dream fulfils a wish, but he does not say "infantile wish"—that will come later. As the journey proceeds, he takes the reader/co-traveller deeper into unconscious wishes. In chapter 5 he finally announces and explores the Oedipus complex. The preoedipal will come with the pitch of investigative excitement in chapter 7, all of which was deliberately expressed in allusions (Freud, 1985d, p. 362); and it is here that Freud seems to associate the deepest investigation into mental processes with a perilous descent into the archaic mother (see Mahony, 1987, pp. 119–110). His stark description is:

> For it must be clearly understood that the easy and agreeable portion of our journey lies behind us. Hitherto, unless I am greatly mistaken, all the paths along which we have travelled have led us towards the light—towards elucidation and fuller understanding. But as soon as we endeavor to penetrate more deeply into the mental process involved in dreaming, every path will end in darkness. [Freud, 1900a, p. 511]

In a word, "corpus" referred to both body and book—an equation later chiselled into the memorable phrase in *Moses and Monotheism*: "The distortion of a text resembles a murder" (Freud, 1939a, p. 43). And so, if the earlier part of Freud's systematic self-analysis led to the discovery of the Oedipus complex and the deceptive power of seductive fantasies, the later part of the self-analysis reshaped those fantasies, in the dream book, into an oedipal and preoedipal exploration of the maternal corpus.

Accordingly, Freud strove for narrative strategy and epistemological investigation to converge in his writing. More than a mere reaction to Fliess's writing failure, Freud's writing cure was an act of self-discovery, self-recovery, and growth—indeed, a self-enabling and self-generative act. [For later examples of self-healing in Freud's writing, see Homans, 1988, pp. 17, 26, 31–33].

Another part of this story is revealing. It deals with the stress that led Freud to wait some six months before taking up the first draft of the *Interpretation of Dreams* and subjecting it to a second and final revision in 1899. [See under the headings "Neurotic symptoms" (pp. 740–741) and "Hysterical symptoms" (p. 736) in the index to Volume 5 of the *Standard Edition*. Cf. Grinstein, 1980, p. 20: some of the repetitiveness in the *Interpretation of Dreams* might have arisen from Freud's "inability to deal adequately with certain unconscious material which, therefore, kept striving for expression during this period. Finally, the working through of infantile attachments, that we now take so much for granted, must have been extremely difficult for him." In the *Interpretation of Dreams*, Freud gave the impression that the work as a whole had been "finished" in 1898 and that he then waited for over a year before deciding to publish it (Freud, 1900a, p. 477; G.W. 2/3: 481). This is simply not true. Freud finished the initial draft by July 1898, and began the second draft in May 1899. Also, as his letters to Fliess show, the second draft underwent revisions and the entirely new seventh chapter was added.] Publicly, Freud attributed the delay in publication to a lack of self-discipline (Freud, 1900a, p. 453) and to an anticipated distress over self-revelation (Freud, 1900a, p. 477). Privately, however, Freud gave Fliess other reasons for not finishing the revision: he could neither fill in the gap left by an important dream that had been dropped, nor could he complete the proposed connections between dreams and neuroses (cf. Freud, 1985d, pp. 318, 332, 338–339, 345). Anzieu's (1975, pp. 594, 619–620, 632, 658, 737–740) historical explanation for the delay in publication manages partially to combine Freud's private and public excuses—namely, the theoretical blockage that held up the revision was underpinned by unconscious fantasies about Freud's own impotence and castration; and these fantasies appeared in dreams that he could not fully verbalize. (Anzieu, 1975, p. 313, even generalizes that a castration fantasy underlay the paralysis that Freud seemed to have experienced before making each of his great discoveries.)

In my opinion, a supplementary explanation is called for, and this involves me in making the first major modification to the title of my presentation. Freud's self-therapy was not just a writing cure—it was also a publishing cure. Much as in our own day—although in his own fashion—Freud was caught in the turmoil of "publish or perish". For him, a complete oedipal victory entailed that he should follow in the steps of Shakespeare and expose his achievement in the public marketplace. Recall that in explaining the Oedipus complex in the *Interpretation of Dreams*, Freud alluded to *Hamlet* as a capital example, and added that the play was written immediately after the death of Shakespeare's father (Freud, 1900a, p. 265). Hence, if the writing of the *Interpretation of Dreams* was Freud's own filial mourning for "the most poignant loss" in his life (Freud, 1900a, p. xxvi), it was concurrently an oedipal triumph by means of a corpus that was both text and mother.

On another front, Freud was resisting full awareness of the degree to which the publication of the *Interpretation of Dreams* would effect an estrangement between himself and Fliess. For all its ills, their friendship had tempered a trying period so that any thought by Freud of a break-up would now be anxiogenic. Besides, in so many ways Freud's relations with Fliess had proved more manageable than those with Breuer—Breuer was strictly a father figure for Freud, whereas Fliess offered the advantageous facility of being turned into a paternal and fraternal transferential object. Moreover, whereas Breuer was reluctant to receive communications about work in progress, Fliess would eagerly receive draft versions from Freud (Freud, 1985d, p. 217). In accordance with such a dynamic, Fliess figured variously in the production of *Interpretation of Dreams*. Let us note, for example, the generative significance proper to Freud's masterpiece: it began with the pregnancy of Freud's wife (the Irma dream) and ended with Freud's rushing its publication so that he could send it on time for Fliess's birthday (Freud, 1985d, pp. 376, 380). Also, if the co-authored *Studies on Hysteria* was Freud's first psychological book, his second was a "Dreamchild" (Freud, 1985, p. 405), which, though singly authored, nevertheless needed Fliess as "godfather" (Freud, 1985d, p. 376).

On balance, however, one must be prepared to accord a whole spectrum of meanings to the composition and publication of the *Interpretation of Dreams*. Freud felt that sending his self-proclaimed dung heap, seedling, and new species (Freud, 1985d, p. 353) to print would arouse "the painful feeling of parting with something which has been one's very own" (Freud, 1985d, p. 376). In sum, Freud symbolically linked the book to the body of himself, his mother, and Fliess—a polyvalency accompanied by separation, castration, and guilt anxieties. Yet I would suggest that the production and release of the *Interpretation of Dreams* constituted primarily an oedipal gesture, however short of complete success. I am thus led to make the second major modification of my presentation: Freud's self-analysis was a writing and publishing cure that was partial, not complete, and the subtext of *The Interpretation of Dreams* constituted a substantial amount of acting out, writing out, and publishing out, whose meanings were insufficiently understood by Freud at the time.

In retrospect, it is easy for us to follow the last act of the amity between Freud and his Berlin colleague—a friendship that was dwindling into a memory. If Freud was desperately asking for a place for dynamic influences in Fliess's dating, Fliess himself was charging that Freud's patients improved or worsened according to strict biological laws (Freud, 1985, p. 159). Freud epitomized their theoretical and personal impasse in this striking formula: "Thus we are becoming estranged from each other through what is most our own" (Freud, 1985d, p. 398). Still, Freud was not quite ready to forsake the bond of writing between them: bound by gratitude, Freud set about writing a kind of diary about one of his patients that he wanted to show

Fliess (Freud, 1985d, p. 388), and he increased his needling of his unproductive friend (Freud, 1985d, pp. 412, 421, 436, 141, 468). By 1901, Freud found himself in an authorial imbroglio: on the one hand, he withdrew the Dora case from publication because he had allegedly lost his "only audience" in Fliess (Freud, 1985d, pp. 450, 456, 457–458 fn.); on the other hand, Freud proposed that together they write a book on bisexuality (pp. 448 and 450). As we know, if that wish were ever fulfilled, it was only in a dream.

When correspondence was circumstantially resumed between Freud and Fliess in 1904, it dealt—not surprisingly—with none other than the subject of publication, and quickly soured into accusations about plagiarism; the very last bitter exchange between Freud and Fliess died out at around the start of the summer holidays. But at the end of those holidays, as we recall, Freud visited the Acropolis; there he experienced a de-realization that was brought on by guilt for surpassing his father, hence a telling residue of Freud's incomplete self-analysis and its writing out. We may now skip to 1936, when it took the celebration for another writer, Romain Rolland, for Freud to write up his Acropolis visit as a piece of self-analysis. In the remaining part of 1936, a ghost from the past would resurrect to put Freud's self-analysis to a gruelling, nightmarish test. Precisely on December 30, Marie Bonaparte wrote to Freud that she had come upon his letters to Fliess and was ready to purchase them from the eager bookseller.

On 3 January 1937, Freud replied that these "most intimate" and "highly embarrassing" letters should not "become known to posterity" (Freud, 1985d, p. 7). Thus, at both ends of his analytics Freud balked at the publication of a piece of his self-analysis—the *Interpretation of Dreams* decades earlier, and now his correspondence with Fliess. But that is not all, although the rest of the story is brief. With the news of his resurrected self-analysis fresh in his mind, Freud sat down two weeks later to write the finished copy of *Analysis Terminable and Interminable* (1937c). (I am relying on my photocopy of the holograph, whose first page bears the date 18.1.1937 also in Freud's handwriting.) The anguishing repercussions of the correspondence continued to remain with him, as can be measured by the fact that prior to 1936 he never talked with his daughter Anna about Fliess, and only "most sparingly" after that date (Freud, 1985d, p. 4). Perhaps from our belated perspective, we can more clearly trace the continuity of the writing cure between *The Interpretation of Dreams* and *Analysis Terminable and Interminable*, and we might even risk summing them in one title: Self-analysis, dreaming, writing: terminable and interminable.

APPENDIX

The dating of Freud's self-analysis is one of the quagmires of psychoanalytic scholarship, not least due to Freud's own erroneous commentary: on 14 November 1897, he wrote that there was no sign of his self-analysis until after the summer holidays (Freud, 1985d, p. 279), a statement belied, for example, by his letters of 22 June (p. 254) and 7 July (p. 255). A further difficulty is that in his correspondence to Fliess, Freud referred to his "self-analysis" as such from 14 August 1897 (p. 261) to 3 January 1899 (p. 338), although his looser allusions to this have fostered a variety of chronological interpretations. With some inconsistencies of his own, Anzieu (1975) breaks it down into three phases:

a. September–October 1897 (pp. 582–583)—but cf. p. 311: "between June and August, 1897, Freud undertakes to make it [his self-analysis] systematic".
b. Spring, 1898, the time when Freud was writing the first version of the *Interpretation of Dreams* (pp. 582–583)—but on page 353 Anzieu assigns the first version to February–July 1898, a dating that is somewhat in agreement with Kris's (Freud, 1954, p. 34) limitation of the first version to the period of the spring and summer, 1898.
c. Spring–summer, 1899, the time of Freud's drafting the second version of the *Interpretation of Dreams* (pp. 582–583)—but in another place Anzieu sees the version beginning in mid-January (p. 370), an alternative that is rather later than autumn 1898, which Kris proposes as the beginning of the second version (1954, p. 34). A greater dating difficulty oc-

curs in Anzieu's irregular chronicling of the third phase of Freud's self-analysis: Freud lived "in a permanent self-analytic atmosphere" (p. 718); his self-analysis ended in 1900 (p. 733), in 1901 (pp. 724, 729); he was in occasional self-analysis from November 1899 to February 1901 (p. 663); his trip to Rome in September 1901 terminated his systematic self-analysis (p. 288).

Although fully assured precision cannot be arrived at, we do have some rectifying facts at our disposal. First, Freud began his dream book in May 1897 (pp. 243 and 249)—that is, before his intensified self-analysis. Second, the current term "systematic self-analysis" must be used with caution: (1) Freud applied a "systematic" analysis to his Irma dream in 1895; (2) nor should "systematic" be used freely to mean uninterrupted, for Freud's systematic self-analysis was in fact one of fits and starts. Evidence will only allow Freud's self-analysis to signify one that was intensified for shorter or longer periods. Equipped with these clarifications, we may conclude the following:

a. Freud tried writing his dream book, quickly encountered a writer's block, and then began a systematic self-analysis. Its first phase was closing towards the end of 1897; on 5 November Freud said that it was trickling (Freud, 1985d, p. 277), and by 14 November he reported its continued interruption (p. 281).
b. The second phase started at around the beginning of December 1897 (pp. 284–285) and culminated in the writing of the four private "dreckological" journals, which were finished by the beginning of February 1898 (p. 301).
c. By 9 February 1898, Freud resumed composing the first version of the dream book (p. 298), which he had begun before the start of his systematic self-analysis; by 7 July 1898 he had finished the first version (p. 319).
d. After a period of fruitful intermittent self-analysis early in 1899 [see the letters of 3 January (p. 338) and 2 March (p. 347)], Freud started composing the second version of the dream book—that is, at the end of May 1899 (p. 353)—and had completed it by 11 September 1899 and saw it published

in November. The ending of this phase of the systematic self-analysis should be left an open question, for relevant traces are intermittent: on 21 December 1899 Freud (p. 392) reported an advance in self-knowledge; on 11 March 1900 he revealed that, with serious matters banished from his mind, he had not written a line for the previous two months (p. 404).

A final caveat: one must take care in interpreting Freud's claim that the writing of the *Interpretation of Dreams* was part of his self-analysis. An initial writer's block had induced Freud to begin a systematic self-analysis. The latter proceeded for some time before Freud got back to writing the *Interpretation of Dreams* proper.

NOTES

1. The dates and places of the Congresses during the period of Freud's self-analysis are as follows: Berlin, September, 1897 (Freud, 1985d, p. 311ff. and 355 ff.); Breslau, December 1897 (ibid., p. 290); possibly in the environs of Vienna, May 1898 (ibid., pp. 314–315); possibly Aussee, July 1898 (ibid., p. 320); Baden, December, 1898 (ibid., p. 337); Innsbruck, April 1899 (ibid., p. 349).
2. I cannot forego making an association to the "separate" categories of the scientific and therapeutic: *science* and *schizo* ultimately come from the same Indo-European root, *skei* (to cut). In Greek, *skhizein* means to split; *science* more immediately stems from the Latin *scire*, to know—that is, to split or separate one thing from another. Thus philological examination unexpectedly sheds light on the possible restorative functions of such different entities as science and schizophrenia.

CHAPTER THREE

From analytic dialogue to published text

Henning Paikin

"Death and life are in the power of the tongue".

Proverbs 18:21

To write and publish case histories is just as important for psychoanalysis and its development as is doing analysis. However, all candidates and analysts have experienced how difficult it is to describe an analytic session in writing. Many misunderstandings among non-analysts concerning psychoanalysis are due to the fact that many case histories that are informative and inspiring for analysts appear as undocumented statements to the reader without psychoanalytic training or without personal experience of the psychoanalytic process. Due to the uniqueness of the analytic process, we can only with difficulty publish the so-called raw data, whatever they may be.

An earlier version of this paper was read before the Fourteenth Nordic Psychoanalytic Congress, Mariehamn, Åland, Finland, August 1994. Previously published in *The Scandinavian Psychoanalytic Review, Vol. 18* (1995).

To report about the analytic experience in writing is still, after 100 years, a challenge for psychoanalysis. The analytic session cannot be told with all its details and nuances, any more than a dream can. And sometimes the details appear just as elusive (cf. Stein, 1988, p. 108; Olinick, 1980, pp. 38, 40).

At the beginning of the first of the *Introductory Lectures*, Freud (1916–17, p. 17) says:

> Nothing takes place in a psycho-analytic treatment but an interchange of words between the patient and the analyst.

And a few sentences later:

> Words were originally magic and to this day words have retained much of their ancient magical power. By words one person can make another blissfully happy or drive him to despair, by words the teacher conveys his knowledge to his pupils, by words the orator carries his audience with him and determines their judgements and decisions.

Taking into consideration Anna O's definition of the treatment, which was the beginning of psychoanalysis, as "the talking cure", and the relevance of the spoken word to the psychoanalytic process, to psychoanalytic supervision, to seminars and conferences, it is surprising how relatively little has been written in the analytic literature, at least in the English language, about speech (exceptions are Spence, 1987; Olinick, 1984; Amati-Mehler, 1993). I dare claim that more is written about silence! How to communicate the psychoanalytic experience, or whether it can be communicated at all, has not received much attention in the analytic literature (Olinick, 1980, p. 37; Haynal, 1993, p. 2).

In this chapter, I will occupy myself mainly with the very limited part of these issues that has to do with the conflict between oral and written exposition. In other words, I will take Freud's words literally: that in the analytic treatment ". . . nothing takes place . . . but an interchange of words", and I will look into the conflict between the spoken and the written word. (I make this choice only to limit the length of my chapter: I am certainly of the opinion that many things happen other than the exchange of words.) I can only hint at other important topics connected with publishing, such as the problems concerning confidentiality and the fact that the analyst, through publishing, places himself in a vulnerable position (see, e.g., Stein, 1988).

Why have analysts been so reluctant to write explicitly about the conflict between orality and literacy that is so central to analytic literature?

I can find two answers: one, that Freud had a unique and unsurpassed literary style, especially in his case histories, which, in an ingenious way, hid the conflict; the other might be that the problems are situated in the borderland between psychoanalysis and many other sciences, such as philology, rhetoric, literary criticism, to mention just a few.

The psychoanalytic dialogue

It is unnecessary to furnish analysts with a detailed description of the prime importance of dialogue in psychoanalytic practice and training. I will therefore only give two examples, as a reminder of the very central and comprehensive position of spoken language within psychoanalysis.

The psychoanalytic process is established by means of spoken communication between analysand and analyst. In analytic work, the analysand's verbal expression has high priority. Other forms of communication are certainly not neglected, but it is standard technique for the analyst to consider it usually (but not always) as his task to verbalize these other pieces of information, whether they are the analysand's gestures, attitudes, actions, affects, or silence! "[T]alking is the method of psychoanalysis", as Fenichel puts it (1946, p. 577). However, talking is also a form of showing. Everything in analysis is both communication and demonstration (Schafer, 1983, p. 222).

I believe that most of us consistently try to get the analysand to communicate with us in oral form. Should the analysand bring letters, diaries or other material, we will usually try to analyse this as resistance. Such material can only be brought into the analysis if the analysand refers to its contents or reads it aloud.

The analytic rationale for this attitude is that language, the spoken word, is a transitional space between psychic reality and physical reality. Most analysts will be of the opinion that language is a tool by means of which we are able to help our analysands. Some might be of the opinion that only carefully verbalized interpretations are helpful, but most analysts today will also take the relationship into consideration. On the other hand, there is hardly an analyst who will dismiss the importance of oral interaction. No analyst will offer analysis by correspondence, although Freud's correspondence with Fliess has been regarded as a kind of analytic process!

Let me emphasize once again that I am not of the opinion that the psychoanalytic process can be reduced to a linguistic interaction. The psychoanalytic process is much more complicated and therefore difficult to describe, especially in writing. This applies especially to those analysands whose difficulties are on a non-verbal, basic-fault level. (A further discussion of these "wordless" analysands would take us too far from the topic.)

The classical analytical setting aims to promote the analysand's oral and spontaneous communication with the analyst, and language is often considered an indifferent tool. Schafer has criticized the opinion that analysands should be able to report their thoughts "freely". Freud made language, especially the *spoken* language, an object of his analysis, but in his technical recommendations he appears to consider it a neutral tool (Schafer, 1992, p. 148).

The dialogue between analysand and analyst is no doubt the primary tool of psychoanalysis. The psychoanalytic dialogue is described so precisely and beautifully by Schafer (1992, p. 156) that I will allow myself a long quotation:

> . . . out of Freud's genius issued an altogether new form of dialogue. He made it possible for therapists and patients to engage in consequential forms of transformational dialogue that have never existed before. He showed therapists how to do things with words to help revise radically their patients' hitherto fixed, unconsciously directed constructions of both subjective experience and action in the world: to use words to change lives in a thought-through, insightful manner. No one before him had done anything as profound, comprehensive, skilful, basically rational and effective. Freud's clinical dialogue alters in crucial ways the analysand's consciously narrated presentation of the self and its history among people.

However, the psychoanalytic dialogue is, as Eiguer (1993, p. 26) emphasizes, also "distinct from all other human dialogues because it is characterized by unpredictability. The analyst listens to the unspeakable, which shocks, indeed disturbs him . . . [one of the] reasons for this unpredictability [is that] the unconscious material is unknown to us".

The psychoanalytic dialogue takes place in privacy but also in a private language, where certain phrases or expressions have a personal, almost metaphorical, meaning that the analyst learns along the way. The more the analysand is able to follow the so-called fundamental rule, the more will the analytic session assume some resemblance to dreams and, in principle, also be interpreted the same way.

The analyst is concerned both with form and content. In most analyses, an idiosyncratic language develops between analysand and analyst in a way similar to the way this happens in all families. The analysand who feels sufficiently safe will also resort to the language of childhood. Amati-Mehler, Argentieri, and Canestri (1993), in their monography on mother tongue and foreign languages, *The Babel of the Unconscious*, pointed out that, in a way, all human beings are polyglots. This means that the adult analysand has, in addition to his normal official daily language, several "languages" at his disposal, depending on the people he talks to—family, children, colleagues, and so on. They write: "every analyst knows how many 'translations' his words and those of his patient require before they become similar words and are able to convey shared meaning" (Amati-Mehler et al., 1993, p. 233). They continue with a quotation from George Steiner, a professor of English and comparative literature, in his major work on translations (Steiner, 1975, p. 47): "Thus, a human being performs an act of translation in the full sense of the word, when receiving a speech–message from any other human being." Poland (1986, p. 257) expresses it in this way: "In trying to express unconscious matters, we use language to approach experience which cannot be exactly reduced to language. . . . Inner experience is not solely verbal. The patient's associations, even at their most free, are already translations. Interpretations, thus, are translations of translations. . . ."

Even Schafer's "action language", which he calls "the native tongue of psychoanalysis" (1976, p. 362), is not to be used directly in the dialogue with the analysand. It is rather ironic that it is still a theoretical language. I believe that the mother tongue of psychoanalysis can only be "heard" in the actual psychoanalytic dialogue between analyst and analysand.

The other example of the oral dialogue's extreme importance in psychoanalysis is supervision or collegiate consultation.

Freud and language

Freud was a master of the spoken and written tongue. "Freud's genius will" according to Kurt Eissler "have to center in his language. . . . ". And Abram Kardiner, who also knew Freud, tells us: "Everything he said was practically fit for print, it was incisive, imaginative, filled with metaphors, analogies and stories, particularly Jewish ones, and it was not wordy. Freud talked like a book" (Mahony, 1982, pp. 3, 9).

Freud's literary style has been the object of detailed studies especially by Mahony (1982, 1984, 1993). In *Freud as a Writer*, Mahony has shown how Freud's certainly not logical style actually recreates much of the analytic situation for the reader. Freud's style is psychoanalytic to an outstanding degree, for it constantly enacts the drive-defence unit (p. 179). It is a unique mixture of primary and secondary processes, and we experience his conscious and unconscious presence (p. 188). His writings blur the boundary between orality and literacy.

It is of interest for our topic that Freud's first book was the neurological treatise *On Aphasia* (1891). Ana-Maria Rizzuto (1993, p. 113), among others, has pointed out that this paper is relevant to Freud's later theorizing and analytic technique. In this treatise, Freud attaches great importance to sound images (Amati-Mehler et al., 1993, p. 30) and in the early works, *The Interpretation of Dreams* (1900a), *The Psychopathology of Everyday Life* (1901b), and *Jokes and Their Relation to the Unconscious* (1905c), he makes use of a long series of rhetoric figures and sound associations in his interpretations: pun, alliteration, rhyme, etc. In other words, it was the *spoken* language that was the object of Freud's analysis. Words in themselves are disconnected and meaningless in the preconscious. They are given coherence, meaning, and intention first by interpretation "In this way the whole domain of verbal wit is put at the disposal of the dreamwork. There is no need to be astonished at the part played by words in dream-formulation. Words, since they are the nodal points of numerous ideas, may be regarded as predestined to ambiguity . . . " (Freud, 1900a, p. 340).

It is amazing that neither Freud himself nor later analysts have, as far as I know, paid attention to the fact that the language Freud placed in the preconscious is the *spoken* language. Written language belongs to consciousness and is a secondary-process activity or, as can be shown, cultural in the historical sense: The spoken language and its distinctive character was "repressed" to the preconscious or unconscious when literacy became dominant. Freud "rediscovered" characteristics of the spoken language through dream interpretation.

Although Freud was a master of language, he was nonetheless

> painfully aware of the limping nature of language as a completely reliable instrument for clinical description. . . . Freud came back again and again to the basic challenge psychic reality poses for exposition: Psychic events are overdeterminated and draw simultaneously from various strata, whereas in verbal exposition these superimposed strata are flattened out into a verbal string; if linearity is the essence of language, superimposition is the keynote of psychic events. [Mahony, 1982, pp. 9, 10]

Freud was explicitly against verbatim reports, as is testified by the following quotations:

> . . . it must be borne in mind that exact reports of analytic case histories are of less value than might be expected. . . . They are, as a rule, fatiguing to the reader and do not succeed in being a substitute for his actual presence at an analysis. [1912e, p. 114]

> Exhaustive verbatim reports of the proceedings during the hours of analysis would certainly be of no help at all. [1918b, p. 13]

In a letter to Jung on 19 April 1908 (Freud/Jung Letters, 1974, p. 141), Freud wrote that a case history story "cannot be narrated but only described". In German it reads: "*ein wirklicher ganzer Fall lässt sich nicht erzählen, nur beschreiben*" (Briefwechsel, 1974, p. 156).

I believe that we can easily agree with Freud, but the problem is that few if any have been able to describe the analytic process as he did.

"To my knowledge", writes Mahony, "no current analyst writer of case histories has insisted as much as Freud on the impossibility of writing a case history" (1993, p. 1033). However, Freud then did the impossible.

A digression on orality

Characteristic conditions for the oral mode can be illustrated by looking at them from a developmental and cultural historical point of view.

The baby is linked to his parents through an actual audiophonic communication system. The mother is able to differentiate the three-week-old baby's cries as expressions of hunger, anger, pain, and so on. The five-week-old baby can distinguish his mother's voice from other voices, though he cannot yet distinguish her face from other faces. It is on the basis of such facts that Anzieu (1979, p. 27) describes a "sound mirror" that exists before the visual mirroring described by Winnicott and Kohut. Anzieu draws attention to the importance of the auditive environments for the early development of the self. (He draws our attention to the fact that the problems of voice and audition have not been of much interest to Freud's commentators, and he calls for research in this area.) This very early prelinguistic root to interpersonal communication makes sense of the fact that the sound of the voice is often more important than the content of what is said. This is especially true when consolation, reassurance, and support are in question, but not only then. It is what Olinick (1982, p. 461) has called "phatic" speech, which has the sole aim of establishing contact. As analysts, we are also accustomed to listening with a "third ear" (Reik, 1951), which, as we all know, means listening to the hidden meanings, but also to the emotional, the unsaid, the unspeakable, or the unthinkable.

It would, of course, be relevant at this point to say something about the development of speech, but that would lead us too far from the topic, so I will not investigate the issue further.

Walter J. Ong, a Professor of Humanities in Psychiatry at Saint Louis University, Missouri, in an already classic work *Orality and Literacy* (1982), has described some primarily oral cultures—that is, cultures without any form of written language—and this is of interest to us. Among other things, Ong emphasizes that the language and the thinking in these cultures are concrete, situational rather than abstract, and that oral personalities, owing to the lack of abstract terms, cannot be introspective. As he puts it: It is hard to talk to yourself for hours on end (p. 34). "Primary orality fosters personality structures that in certain ways are more communal and externalized and less introspective than those common among literates. Oral communication unites people in groups. Writing and reading are solitary activities . . ." (p. 69). Speech unites, even when one speaker approaches a large audience!

In oral cultures, people do not say anything that has no meaning or actuality for the speaker and the listener; writing is a different instance since it preserves everything. Memory is short in oral cultures—one knows only what can be recalled: ". . . oral memory differs significantly from textual memory in that oral memory has a high somatic component. . . . The oral word . . . never exists in a simply verbal context, as the written word does. Spoken words are always modifications of a total, existential situation, which always engages the body" (Ong, 1982, p. 67).

This summary of some aspects of primitive oral cultures is no doubt akin to what we know from the psychoanalytic dialogue, which aims among other things at bringing the analysand into the oral universe by verbalizing his thoughts. The analytical dialogue is, like other oral dialogues, mutual, actual, infinite, and creates mutual experience and includes more than words (Ong, 1982, p. 101). Thus, it gives a special admission to the preconscious (and unconscious), which no written communication can do. Psychic change begins when, in the presence of the analyst, the analysand says aloud what he hardly dares to think.

Ong (1982, p. 71) mentions, as Fink also does (1993), some physical characteristics of sound. Sound tells us about the interior of things, whereas sight only registers the surface. The expression on the face of a human being tells us something about his inner life, but facial expression can be controlled much better than the voice. People who are in acoustic contact with each other know something about each other's interior. We are in the hands of one another as far as the oral sphere is concerned.

Fink describes it in this way: "A spoken word will only linger on for a fraction of a second before becoming past. It may stay consciously or unconsciously in the mind of the patient and analyst, but it will be subject to emotionally determined change and possible distortion. It will never again be the same as when it was spoken" (p. 15).

From dialogue to retelling

The other example of the importance of oral dialogue in psychoanalysis is, as mentioned, supervision.

Let me give two very short but typical vignettes:

A supervisee looked up from his notes and said: "I really don't know whether it was I or the patient who said this."

Another supervisee, who had given an excellent report about a session, added with all the signs of guilt that the report was a "fake", because it was continuous and meaningful, which she didn't think was the case in the session.

Both of these vignettes can be interpreted in many different ways, but I am sure they illustrate the discrepancy between the analyst's experience and the retelling. That the same applies for analysands was nicely illustrated to me once by an analysand who kept a diary of his analysis. The analysand realized that notes concerning "important insights" were not recognizable a few months later, and he could not understand why he had made these notes as they no longer appeared important to him.

Although the supervisee depends on his written notes, supervision is a dialogue in which the supervisee's spontaneous presentation is, with some approximation, used in a way similar or parallel to the analytic situation. Supervision can nowadays take place by telephone, but even then it is an oral dialogue.

Olinick has pointed out (1980, p. 39) that the psychoanalyst's skills are primarily developed through oral communication and its non-verbal concomitants. Auditory and introspective channels are emphasized. However, memory, fantasy, and imagination exist largely in visual terms. Consequently, the subjective recording and the objective reporting of intrapsychic and interpersonal events of the psychoanalytic situation are handicapped by the need to make use of modalities that are relatively unnatural and unfamiliar. By borrowing a phrase from Aldous Huxley, Olinick asks what is the "adequate verbal equivalent" for the affective quality of a patient's silence?

I am fully in agreement with Tuckett (1994, p. 1182), when he writes: "What is to be communicated seemed there to us at the time, but we will all have had the frustrating experience of trying to tell someone else about it and discovering that what we say sounds much less convincing than it felt in the session, when it was formulated. (Bion makes the interesting point . . . that even the notes we take . . . often seem baffling or unconvincing to us later.)"

We know from supervision how the so-called report of a single session attains a similarity to the telling of the manifest dream where the dreamer can continue to make additions and commentaries because the dream was so ambiguous (Stein, 1988, p. 112). The above two vignettes illustrate how the telling of a session is a process similar to the secondary revision of dreamwork. And as there is only one dreamer who is responsible for the dream, so there is only one analyst who is responsible for his version of the "manifest" analytical dialogue the "latent" meanings of which we can try to discover and discuss. Concerning this issue, Tuckett (1994, p. 1184) writes: "The central point of a psychoanalytic process is that it cannot rely on rational verbalization alone, and in his attempt to communicate, the analyst *says* more than he consciously knows. This is a strength, not a weakness . . . " (see also Spence, 1987, p. 174). A strength, yes, when the analyst *speaks about* the analytical process with one or several colleagues, because in an oral dialogue the participating listener will have the opportunity to make a trial identification with the reporting analyst and possibly point out countertransference elements.

Psychoanalysis is today a well-established, independent science that presents some *technical* difficulties, like other sciences, for instance history and mathematics (the examples are not chosen at random!). Historians must, just like us, hear or read reports about events that have to be combined, interpreted, and retold in light of the historian's assumptions. What the historian publishes is his own version of the facts. The psychoanalytic story is a retelling of the analysand's telling: the amount of detail must be extremely reduced and condensed. We cannot and should not be more precise than the historians. If the details were not reduced, a hypothetically "complete" telling should contain the analysand's "whole" prehistory, everything the analysand said, thought, or might have thought and so on, and the same applies for the analyst. (See Haynal, 1993, p. 3, for similar viewpoints.) If I have understood Spence (1982) correctly, he originally suggested something of the kind, although he later changed his mind (Spence, 1987).

The use of the tape-recorder demands a more thorough discussion than can be given within the limits of this chapter. It is, however, obvious that a tape-recording can only reproduce the words—that is, a very limited part of the manifest material—but it describes neither the comprehensive unconscious communication between analysand and analyst nor, of course, the analyst's countertransference.

We need not have a different attitude towards the analyst's report of a session than to the report of the manifest dream: it is the starting point for our investigation. It is, after all, the "latent"—that is, the unconscious—coherence and meaning that is of importance.

One more digression: writing is a technology

Speech is a natural human potential, which develops as an integrated part of the child's maturation and development; writing, however, is a technology, which can only be taught at a much later time. Written language has in many ways a status other than speech as far as psychology and cognition are concerned: It is context-free, autonomous, and one of the preconditions for abstract thinking. Writing implies consciousness and also increases consciousness and internalization. In contrast to speech, writing is a lonely occupation. The process of writing implies, for better or for worse, a distance from the material. The written text attempts to be logical and precise and will therefore be somewhat circumstantial, whereas the spoken word is always part of a total situation and does not appear merely as words. In a text, the words stand alone. The living word becomes dead on paper if it is not, incidentally, written by a brilliant writer. As analysts, we can listen with the third ear, but we cannot write with a third hand!

Historically, the development has been such that written language has influenced spoken language to the extent that the oral tradition no longer exists, except within the precincts of psychoanalysis (also mentioned by Olinick, 1984, p. 614). Most often, we regard writing only as an assistance to memory, but in Plato's dialogue "Phaedros", Socrates recounts a myth where the point is that the inventor of alphabetic writing is told that instead of being an aid to memory and wisdom, writing will be a tool for forgetfulness. As analysts, we know very well that this is true, and this is one of the reasons why we usually do not require notes about our analysands. We have experienced that we can recall what is analytically relevant, and we know our analysands better than our relatives, about whom we do not need notes! From supervisions, we know that what makes sense in a session will be remembered or will be recalled during the supervision. We also advise our analysands not to write down the manifest dream, because it will only be a "tertiary revision", which will not ease admission to the latent dream-thoughts.

There are also aspects of writing that might be frightening and take on a superego quality. The written word is in the nature of an oracle: it is separated from its author, and the paradox is that although the written word is dead, it lives an "eternal" life of its own, because it will survive even if it is disproved! From this, it follows that the writer never knows how his text will be read by his colleagues. "The writer's audience is always a fiction" (Ong, 1982, p. 101).

These factors no doubt contribute to many analysts' reluctance to publish cases. Another factor I have already focused on is, of course, that the psychoanalytic process involves the analyst personally.

From retelling to text

Even the characterization of the analytic process gives rise to delicate questions: Is it to be understood as a report, a description, a story, a narration, a translation, or a transcription? Many more definitions can be considered, but these examples amply illustrate that the answer will depend on the analyst's metascientific point of view, artistic talent, choice of literary genre, and understanding of the difference between speech and writing.

The distance between psychoanalytic dialogue and analytic literature has always been great. I have already mentioned some of the reasons for this: It is difficult, perhaps impossible, to verbalize the regressive, ambiguous, non-verbal, emotional, and intimate character of the psychoanalytic process. This is also due to the fact that while the analyst is listening, he is also trying to register the process, the latent messages of the analysand and his own emotional reactions and fantasies, at one and the same time. Being difficult in itself, it is not possible to describe it as a dream or, in Fenichel's words, it: ". . . can only be reproduced in words inexactedly, always with the addition of 'something like' . . ." (Fenichel, 1939, p. 10). We can therefore well understand why many analysts in their case reports resort to abstract metapsychological concepts.

Sandler (1983, p. 35) has emphasized that the "official" or "public" formulation of psychoanalytical terms has multiple, context-dependent meanings. At the same time, he has indicated that the practising analyst has his private, preconscious, implicit theories, which function well in his daily work, even if there are possible self-contradictions. These two matters contribute considerably to the gulf between the living, multiple-layered psychoanalytic dialogue and the manner of its presentation for publication.

Consideration for the confidentiality of the analysand is often mentioned as the reason for the reluctance analysts have shown to publish their case histories. I will not delve any further into this problem, which is self-evident. Instead I will repeat that the written—that is, the published—word is somewhat frightening. It is out of the author's control, and it lives forever. It cannot be changed or annulled. Furthermore, there are superego-coloured fantasies about how the text will be read and interpreted by kind or not so kind colleagues. The problems concerning discretion are greater for the author than for the analysand, whose identity can be disguised. But any case history worth reading tells us quite a lot about the analyst, whether he wishes it or not: that is a price we have to pay.

No wonder, then, that so few have attempted to publish more comprehensive cases. The editors of *The International Journal of Psycho-Analysis* issued an invitation to send in such cases—an invitation that must have reached at least 7000 analysts worldwide. In reply, they received only 26 manuscripts (!), of which 15 were published (Tuckett, 1991, p. 377).

Conclusion

Notwithstanding the absolutely central position of oral dialogue in psychoanalysis, we cannot do without the published text; we need text, both for theorizing and for case histories. Without written sources, we would not be able to communicate and discuss internationally and over time. We would not even be able to think abstractly. And we also need to publish in order to communicate psychoanalysis to other professionals and interested lay people.

In this chapter, I have tried to focus on some of the difficulties and conflicts that occur in translating the analytic dialogue and process to public text. The question is whether, or how, these difficulties can be overcome. One tentative answer could be as follows.

As psychoanalysis is an interpretive and not an empirical science, every single case will have several different versions. Just as the manifest dream always has more than a single true interpretation, so the analytic session, too, has more than a single true version. Just as there is only one dreamer who is responsible for the dream, so there is only one narrator or writer who is responsible for *his* version of the analytic dialogue. There are always several possible versions: a tape-recording will present one version; the analysand will give another; and the analyst will certainly give a third version. Similarly, the analyst's published version, actually co-authored by the analysand, will be interpreted in various ways by different readers. The author's version is not the final one.

The difficulties involved in transforming the analytic dialogue into text are great, but may in principle not be so different from those encountered in transforming other similar, intense, emotional, and significant human experiences. What is the "*adequate verbal equivalent*" of, let us say, falling in love? The answer is only to be found in poetry and literature. And although a case history is not fiction in the pedestrian meaning of the word, every case history is a narrative that can be interpreted and with which we can establish a dialogue. If we take *an analytic attitude*—that is, an interpretative attitude—both dialogue and narration are only starting points for our analytic activity. Put in a somewhat more provocative manner: the publishing analyst and his reader are perhaps in the same boat.

There are, of course, differences between the oral analytic dialogue and an imagined dialogue with a text. The most essential difference is, however, that the analysand can change, and so can the reader, but the text itself, in terms of printed matter, remains unaltered. Otherwise, the dialogue and the principles of interpretation are the same.

What I have focused on in this paper are *some* of the *technical* difficulties involved in communicating the analytic session and process. These difficulties certainly explain in part why so few analysts have published more comprehensive case histories. The difficulties are, however, only a relative hindrance for writing, since the text becomes in itself the object of the reader's interpretation. The dialogue and the process continue.

CHAPTER FOUR

Writing in psychoanalysis

Antonio Alberto Semi

The theme of writing in psychoanalysis is at once clearly delimited and quite broad. However, before dealing with the more specific question of this main focus, I would like to make a few observations on the broader issue of writing—that is, the problems that writing itself, from its very origins, has posed for mankind. It must have been a truly ecstatic moment when man understood that a concrete fact—a mark on a tablet or a rock, a carving on a tree—could be linked to a thought. No activity is more consistently symbolic than writing, and no activity more consistently recalls the original reality of the symbol, in both its material and its psychic make-up.

Narrowing the field, I will give only two examples drawn from our two main cultural roots: ancient Greece and Judaism. Indeed, these two cultures—or some of their important representatives—have dealt, in quite different ways, with the problems and possibilities offered by writing.

The classic reference point of the Greek tradition is a text by Plato on writing. I have taken the liberty of citing it at length because at least two passages concern us quite closely. In the first, Socrates, according to Plato, tells Phaedrus (in the dialogue of the same name) the following story:

> At the Egyptian city of Naucratis, there was a famous old god, whose name was Theuth; the bird which is called the Ibis is sacred to him, and he was the inventor of many arts, such as arithmetic and calculation and geometry and astronomy and draughts and dice, but his great discovery was the use of letters. Now in those days the god Thamus was the king of the whole country of Egypt; and he dwelt in that great city of Upper Egypt which the Hellenes call Egyptian Thebes, and the god himself is called by them Ammon. To him came Theuth and showed his inventions, desiring that the other Egyptians might be allowed to have the benefit of them; he enumerated them, and Thamus enquired about their several uses. . . . But when they came to letters, This, said Theuth, will make the Egyptians wiser and give them better memories; it is a specific both for the memory and for the wit. Thamus replied: O most ingenious Theuth, the parent or inventor of an art is not always the best judge of the utility or inutility of his own inventions to the users of them. And in this instance, you who are the father of letters, from a paternal love of your own children have been led to attribute to them a quality which they cannot have; for this discovery of yours will create forgetfulness in the learners' souls, because they will not use their memories; they will trust to the external written characters and not remember of themselves. The specific which you have discovered is an aid not to memory, but to reminiscence, and you give your disciples not truth, but only the semblance of truth; they will be hearers of many things and will have learned nothing; they will appear to be omniscient and will generally know nothing; they will be tiresome company, having the show of wisdom without the reality. ["Phaedrus", 274–275]

This is the first passage: it is radically contrary to the idea that wisdom—which is to say true knowledge—can be acquired through reading. It is noteworthy here that Plato shifts the focus from the discovery of writing to its use. In a certain sense, then, this well-known passage strays from our theme, so to speak: it concerns readers more than writers. But further on there is another short piece that concerns us more directly. Socrates poses to Phaedrus an analogy between sowing and the transmission of knowledge: writing is compared to the "gardens of Adonis", small pots in which seeds germinate rapidly but die in eight days. True sowing is, instead, linked to oral transmission. Socrates, however, points out that

> . . . in the *garden of letters* [the philosopher] will sow and plant, but only for the sake of recreation and amusement; he will write them down as memorials to be treasured against the forgetfulness of old age, by himself, or by any other old man who is treading the same path. He will rejoice in beholding their tender growth. ["Phaedrus", 276; italics added]

The first excerpt, we could venture, represents the relational point of view, the second, the intrapsychic.

The other cultural root of our problem is Judaism. It is interesting to note that in classical Greek culture it is a written text, on the topic of writing, that praises the oral transmission of knowledge, whereas in Judaism reflections on writing relied for many centuries upon oral tradition. Only in the first centuries of the Vulgar era were these reflections collected in the *Mishnah* and still later in the *Talmud.* In the Hebrew tradition it is said that God gave two laws to Moses upon the Sinai, the written law and the oral law. It is this twofold nature of the law that attributes value to the blank spaces, between the letters and between the lines, of the written law. Without dwelling on questions of Jewish mysticism, however, I would like to emphasize two elements of the Judaic contribution to the problems of writing. The first concerns contents: writing serves first and foremost to deliver the Law. The second element is striking and has been the subject of many Midrashim: the Law was given upon the Sinai to a person, Moses, who had a speech defect. It is written:

> And Moses spake before the Lord, saying, "Behold, the children of Israel have not hearkened unto me; how then shall Pharaoh hear me, who am of uncircumcised lips?" [Ex., 6.12]

Shortly thereafter it continues:

> And the Lord said unto Moses, "See, I have made thee a god to Pharaoh: and Aaron thy brother shall be thy prophet.

> Thou shalt speak all that I command thee: and Aaron thy brother shall speak unto Pharaoh, that he send the children of Israel out of his land." [Ex., 7.1–2]

Aaron, of course, possesses a long rod that turns into a snake, eating other snakes and moistening the land it touches. Aaron is also the one who will enter into the promised land, while Moses can only look at it. What interests me here, however, is the symbolic personification in Moses of the incompleteness of the word and the distinction that is drawn between those who (like Aaron) deliver the law and the commands of God orally, and those who, instead, receive it and write it down. Thus, just as the blank spaces on the written page take on meaning, so the difference between Moses and Aaron—between the person who carries a written text and the one who formulates it verbally in an intelligible form—represents a difference in the state of thought, which I will try to describe later.

I don't believe I can take these scholarly analyses any further, but I would like to point out a possible analogy between the Platonic reference to writing as play and the figures of Moses and Aaron. In both cases, we could say, the element of solitude is in the foreground. In Plato's case it is the life-giving, playful qualities of solitude that are stressed; in Moses and Aaron the accent falls on the element of inefficacy and yet of truth. The fact remains that, in both cultures, the word, in order to effectively transform others, must follow certain rules: those of the dialogues and symposia among philosophers in the first case and those of language in the latter. The word of the text is ineffectual if it is not spoken.

Before closing these historical observations, however, I would like to point out a relative timelessness, or a relative constant, if I may be allowed the oxymoron. There is no need to emphasize that this ancient debate concerns us directly, since one of the issues of psychoanalytic writing is whether it can serve to transmit psychoanalysis. But is it possible to transmit knowledge through writing? Or, what is meant by knowledge in our case? Or, more simply, is the transmission of knowledge possible *only* through writing? Or, lastly, is it possible to transmit knowledge *only* orally?

It is obvious that I am concerned with the inaugural moments of writing. Thus, a third observation on the birth of writing might help highlight one of the two elements that the Hebrew root gives us: that of the Law, and thus of power.

One man witnessed the zero degree of writing: he had the chance to observe a group of people begin, if not to write, at least to understand the significance of writing. This person was Claude Lévi-Strauss, who wrote about it in *A World on the Wane* (1961, ch. 25: "A Writing Lesson"). While studying the Nambikwara, an Amazonian tribe unfamiliar with writing, he handed out pieces of paper and pencils to some tribe members. The chief observed Lévi-Strauss (who was also the chief of his group) taking notes during the interviews, and he began scrawling long wavy lines on the paper in response to the anthropologist's questions. However, except to discuss some "clarifications" when Lévi-Strauss asked him, the tribal chief refused to say what he had written (which, of course, was non-existent). Then he began to use the pieces of paper to issue commands to his own small tribe and demonstrate his power. Lévi-Strauss comments,

> So the Nambikwara had learnt what it meant to write! But not at all, as one might have supposed, as the result of a laborious apprenticeship. *The symbol had been borrowed, but the reality remained quite foreign to them.* Even the borrowing had had a sociological, rather than an intellectual object: for it was not a question of knowing specific things, or understanding them, or keeping them in mind, but merely of enhancing the prestige and authority of one individual—or one function—at the expense of the rest of the party. A native, still in the period of the stone age, had realized that even if he could not himself understand the great instrument of understanding he could at least make it serve other ends. [p. 290; italics added]

In a rapid excursus on the history of writing, Lévi-Strauss then argues that ". . . nothing of what we know of writing, or of its role in evolution (p. 291)" justifies an "intellectual" conception of the origin of writing. On the contrary, ". . . when writing makes its début . . . it seems to favour rather the exploitation than the enlightenment of mankind" (p. 292). Archaeologists studying the third millennium—the age of the birth of cuneiform writing—agree on this thesis. Writing arises with the Law, or, if we wish, with a social organization meant to exploit large masses of individuals:

> . . . the use of writing for disinterested ends and with a view to satisfactions of the mind in the fields either of science or the arts, is a secondary result of its invention—and may even be no more than a way of reinforcing, justifying, or dissimulating its primary function. [p. 292]

I believe that this reference to a primary/secondary category is applicable to our writing as well: we assume our responsibility for attempting to broaden the secondary outcome while remaining aware of the fact that, in the act of writing, we are also dealing with our inner savage or inner child at play with bows and arrows. (Freud, 1900a).

Returning to the problem at hand, we must first of all observe that, if writing in psychoanalysis is already difficult, then writing about writing psychoanalysis is even more so. My discussion of the problem will begin—as we are wont to do, somewhat superstitiously, religiously, and, lastly, scientifically—with the writings of Freud. Observations on writing can be found in a number of Freud's texts and in particular in some letters. When I first began reflecting on the topic, I thought of starting off with one of two texts written for publication: either the early writings on hysteria, or the introductory chapter to the case of the Wolf Man (Freud, 1918b [1914]). The first instance, I thought, offered the advantage of allowing us to observe an inaugural situation that, to a certain though lesser degree, all of us have had to face (if for no other reason than to write up the case histories needed to become associate members). In the second instance, on the other hand, Freud had already made fundamental contributions to the study of the human soul and, as was his habit, tossed a stone into the pond of ideas, polemically addressing a fundamental problem: the relevance that writing in psychoanalysis has for the transmission of psychoanalytic knowledge.

> I am unable to give either a purely historical or a purely thematic account of my patient's story; I can write a history neither of the treatment nor of the illness, but I shall find myself obliged to combine the two methods of presentation. It is well known that no means has been found of in any way introducing into the reproduction of an analysis the sense of conviction which results from the analysis itself. Exhaustive verbatim reports of the proceedings during the hours of

> analysis would certainly be of no help at all; and in any case the techniques of the treatment make it impossible to draw them up. So analyses such as this are not published in order to produce conviction in the minds of those whose attitude has hitherto been recusant and sceptical. The intention is only to bring forward some new facts for investigators who have already been convinced by their own clinical experiences. [Freud, 1918b [1914], p. 13]

Here, then, the import of writing is greatly reduced. Freud clearly affirms the point that one is writing for insiders, those who are already convinced of the psychoanalytic method. It is interesting that he poses the problem not in terms of scientific demonstration, but in terms of rhetorical efficacy and the degree of persuasiveness that psychoanalytic writing can have. This degree is, in fact, close to zero. Freud issued these warnings within the context of his disagreement with Jung and Adler, after having recognized that the resistances to psychoanalysis had shifted. At first, these had been expressed in the pure and simple negation of the existence of psychoanalytic phenomena. The dispute with Jung and Adler, instead, had the novel feature that the phenomena were not negated, but interpreted in a reductive or at any rate partial manner, incompatible with the entire theoretic corpus elaborated up to that moment (Freud, 1914).

I believe that these questions on resistance to psychoanalysis must still be kept in mind (in the context, of course, of present-day reality) by those of us who publish a journal of psychoanalysis—a journal that, by its very nature, is directed not only at members of our own psychoanalytic community but at all its interested readers. What resistances do these readers have? What is resistance to psychoanalysis like nowadays? How many of our readers still belong to those whom I call (to myself) the "pot of soup types"? [It may be recalled that Freud, in Lecture XXIX of the *New Introductory Lectures on Psycho-Analysis*, 1933a [1932], noted, "But if you ask how much of dream-interpretation has been accepted by outsiders—by the many psychiatrists and psychotherapists who warm their pot of soup at our fire (incidentally without being very grateful for our hospitality) . . . —the reply gives little cause for satisfaction" (p. 8). If this sentence contains, as I think it does, an allusion to the witch's kitchen scene in Goethe's *Urfaust*, then those doing the cooking are the bogeys.]

And how many, instead, have an interest in psychoanalysis? To write psychoanalysis—which is neither "describing psychoanalysis" nor "writing about psychoanalysis"—in the attempt, through the act of writing, to accomplish an act of persuasion (in the most noble sense of the word), runs the risk of attempting an impossible task. And what is the sense of persuading?

We can describe several facets of this impossible, yet very real task (like analysis itself), beginning with the psychic functions necessary for writing, writing as a combination of functions necessary for psychoanalytic elaboration, and the description of the other, the stranger (or the reader in this case), and the vicissitudes of the writer–reader pair. I wonder if, in this sense, the editorial board–author relationship is not to the author–reader relationship as analysis is to the relationship between the patient and a significant figure in his past. I ask myself this question and immediately reply in the negative, not because this is not true, but because there can be no working context, no setting, or no framework for analysing this relationship. Still, I wonder.

These questions are even more pertinent in a broader context: for instance, no novels are written in Italian any longer. As we know, this incapacity or impossibility has cultural origins; in other countries, such as Germany, the United States, England, or Israel, there are still outstanding novelists. Italy, however, has a novel-writing crisis. Therefore, we might also ask ourselves whether this does not also concern, albeit in a particular form, the paucity of satisfactory clinical articles. In other words, the specific crisis of individuality and subjectivity that is moving across our culture could take on a particular form in our country, reflected both in the "novel-writing crisis" and in clinical psychoanalytic writing. The editorial board, then, would find itself faced with a reflection—in the visual sense of the word—of something that lies beyond and proves to be an unsurmountable limitation.

As far as Freud is concerned, we should first consider a well-known observation from the introduction to the second edition of *The Interpretation of Dreams* (1900a). I believe that an important variant of our problem is to be found here. (It bears emphasizing, though, that this was written well after *Studies on Hysteria*, 1895d). We can suppose that the personal element in those writings was much less conscious than we think of in rereading them today. At any rate, in the preface Freud writes very simply, "This book has a further subjective significance for me personally—a significance which I only grasped after I had completed it" (p. XXVI). He is referring to his reaction to his father's death. *The Interpretation of Dreams* is, as we know, also a lengthy working-through of his relationship with his father. And Freud's relationship with his father, to suggest a connection with the quote from Lévi-Strauss, also involves power. But what interests me here is the fact that only *after* writing it was Freud able to think clearly about this fact.

What is the nature, then, of a process that expresses a thought, unknown to the author, by means of thoughts that have been elaborated at length and with difficulty? This question leads us from a relational to an intrapsychic level to query whether, in investigating the latter, the question of writing psychoanalysis for publication does not take on another meaning.

In addition to the texts written for publication, we are also well acquainted with Freud's letters; these contain a number of observations, at times confession-like disclosures, about Freud's writing. An example is the letter of 3 December 1897, to Fliess. This letter is of great interest because it compares Freud's difficulty in writing at that time both to a dream in which he was in Rome, walking the streets and surprised that the street and shop signs were in German, and to his difficulty in getting to Rome, linked to his infatuation "for the hero worship of the Semitic Hannibal". But let us look at the description of his difficulty in writing:

> Probably it was not an auspicious day, however; the new idea which occurred to me in my euphoria retreated, no longer pleased me, and is now waiting to be born again. Every now and then ideas dart through my head which promise to realize everything, apparently connecting the normal and the pathological, the sexual and the psychological problem, and then they are gone again and I make no effort to hold onto them because I indeed know that neither their disappearance nor their appearance in consciousness is the real expression of their fate. On such quiet days as yesterday

> and today, however, everything in me is very quiet, terribly lonely, I cannot talk about it to anyone, nor can I force myself to work, deliberately and voluntarily as other workers can. I must wait until something stirs in me and I become aware of it. And so I often dream whole days away. [p. 284]

As can be seen, daydreaming takes the place of writing, though it is certainly less fruitful.

Writing, in its actuality, is strictly bound to solitude, and when one is unable to write one experiences a different kind of solitude, in which "all is silence and terrible loneliness". I will return to this point below. From this passage and others it is apparent that Freud wrote in spurts, when he felt that the pressure within him had reached the end of its gestation, the right moment for its release. Freud experienced periods in which he was incapable of elaborating anything, which alternated with others in which his ideas linked together, building *Auffassungen*[1] that became highly persuasive to him and subjectively true.

Then it would happen that, in writing, these ideas appeared to be lost, and perhaps the writing just lay there, incomplete or unable to be completed. At length, in a new burst, he would sit down again at his desk and rewrite the work. An entire space had to be recovered and filled between the "vision"—of which he spoke explicitly as early as 1895—and his other writings. ["During an industrious night last week, when I was suffering from that degree of pain which brings about the optimal condition for my mental activities, the barriers suddenly lifted, the veils dropped, and everything became transparent—from the details of the neuroses to the determinants of the consciousness" (letter, 20 October 1895, p. 146). He adds, "only in attempting to report it to you . . . the whole matter became obvious to me".] The difficulty lies in the shift from fantasy to writing and to scientific writing. (At any rate, Freud often speaks of the connection between fantasy and scientific creativity, as, for example, when he speaks of the metapsychological "witch".) Here Freud points out something about the function of writing that I would like to dwell on: this is the bridging function between two representational systems, which, in my opinion—and also as described by him—exists between the systems *Pcs.* and *Cs.* and not between the *Ucs.* and the *Pcs.* The first system is one of both thing- and word-representations, typical of the *Pcs.*; the other qualifies the *Cs.* and concerns word-representations only. Freud says little about the censorship between these two systems, although at the end of chapter 7 of *The Interpretation of Dreams* (1900a) he indicates its importance. The whole of chapter 6 of the same work also seems to be devoted to the fundamental description of how the *Cs* can accommodate configurations of thought that are characteristic of the *Ucs.*

In the metapsychological essays, attention is mostly centred on developing an explanation of the unconscious system's rules and on the transition between unconscious and preconscious. But, as we know, from then on Freud was reluctant to speak about the functioning of the barrier between *Pcs* and *Cs.* [Note, for example, the fact that one of the "lost" essays that was to constitute *Metapsychology* was devoted to consciousness (C. L. Musatti, Introduction to *Opere di Sigmund Freud*, vol. 8, pp. XI ff.) and the editor's note to *Metapsicologia* (ibid., p. 3). There remains, however, the important treatment of Section 6 of the essay on "The Unconscious" (Freud, 1915e) and the further references, identified in the notes. For the characteristics of the "conscious", for the description of ways of becoming conscious, and for its role in constructing the theory, see *An Outline of Psycho-Analysis* (1940a [1938]), which contains a great many observations on this subject, often made in reference or in passing. For a more systematic description, although this, too, for the purpose of developing the description of the unconscious, see *Beyond the Pleasure Principle* (1920g, esp. ch. 4) and *The Ego and the Id* (1923b).] Also, as late as 1938, in *An Outline of Psycho-Analysis* (1940a [1938]), Freud was to state "the starting-point for this investigation is provided by a fact without parallel, which defies all explanation or description—the fact of consciousness" (p. 157).

However, our task here is to observe, investigate, and discuss an activity belonging to that very system (after the introduction of the second hypothesis, this activity is even more difficult to investigate).

Up to this point, I have attempted to illustrate several fundamental issues about writing in general and in psychoanalysis in particular. Thus we have looked at the *auxiliary characteristics* of writing (mentioned by Plato), the *symbolic characteristics*, expressing relationships of power, connected to the Law and the father (through Moses, Freud, and a Nambikwara chieftain), *the need for material solitude*, and *the need for an inner permeability* that acts as a safeguard against loneliness. But we have also observed the existence of a *relational aspect*, between author and reader, and another, more specific one, between author and, shall we say, the psychoanalytic journal as a group. This has allowed us to glimpse a critical condition that goes beyond our immediate scope, belonging, as it does, to our times and pertaining to the difficulty in the constitution of the subject—or of a new way of being subjects—in our culture. We should note also that this is an obvious contradiction, since something as exquisitely individual as subjectivity is manifestly codified, in all its possible modalities, by culture.

I will now add another probative element to this consideration: a great many of the manuscripts that are sent to the *Rivista* are not conceived primarily for print but are intended for presentation at meetings between colleagues (Institutes, Congresses, etc.); only later do they become articles. Sometimes it happens that the greatest resistance encountered by the editorial board occurs when the author is asked to change the style of his text from that of an oral presentation to that of an article. On some occasions it has been objected that it is not permissible to interfere with personal style—a sacrosanct objection, provided we do not confuse style with genre.

I would like to attempt a definition of some symptomatic characteristics of this conduct. Compared to writing an article, oral communication, such as a paper given at a Congress or read to a group of colleagues, may present less difficulty for some, while others find it more difficult. The proper compilation of a bibliography, the accuracy in quoting a text, the straightening up of grammar and syntax would seem to be for many a vile task. We can modify the guidelines for authors to make them clearer and simpler but I do not believe that this is where the problem lies. On the one hand, the rigid rules of written language—which, however, become more elastic and yielding the more one uses them—cannot be disregarded past a certain point (e.g. correct syntax and vocabulary). On the other hand, we cannot fail to observe certain conventions or norms according to which the boundary between quotation and plagiarism is established through the use of conventional elements, such as quotation marks and the page number that the passage is quoted from. But our authors are all persons with a long experience of studying and reading; if only by reading, they must have learned not only how to write, but also how to recognize the rules that govern it. No, that is not the problem. The problem is that the other person, the addressee of communication, is present during the oral communication and absent when we are writing. An author writes for himself and does not need to verify (for himself) the origin of an excerpt he is quoting: he knows that he knows it. The problem, then, arises from the fact that the written communication—since writing, even if it is not meant to be read, is a form of communication—must be precise in order to convey even a limited effect. But what does "precise" mean?

I think all of us have on occasion scribbled a note for fear of forgetting a dream, part of a therapeutic session, or something we had to buy, and we have done it in an evocative manner rather than in detail. Likewise, I think it has happened at one time or another that we have then been unable to reconstruct exactly the sequence of that session or have found ourselves staring blankly at four hastily scrawled words, unable to overcome repression.

Writing with clarity should prevent this from happening. We cannot expect the power of evocation to be completely preserved, and we must acknowledge that repression proper has perhaps been substituted by the repression of the affect. The effort is worth making, however, since this may render certain contents, otherwise forever lost to consciousness, accessible, as Freud, too, reminds us concerning negation (1925h).

The fact is that the *Cs* is part of the ego, but it functions according to its own rules. For example, it does not have its own mnemic systems; the representations it receives can enter consciousness because, on the one hand, they are afforded attention (a little-studied function). On the other hand, other functions—pertaining to another system—contribute to the creation of representations by cathecting traces deposited in the various mnemic systems. It is not without significance, then, that reading is a system that uses visual perceptions to induce word representations and that writing constitutes the translation of sets of word representations into visually perceptible material signs. We could perhaps say that writing is a substitutive activity by means of which the ego devises an artificial memory for the *Cs*. The theory is not new, but it deserves reconsideration, if we clarify that in this instance attention must be projected outward and activate perception, and that affects and representations once again go different ways.

Come on now, it could be objected, what are you getting at? What secret can be unveiled through the study of writing, and of psychoanalytic writing in particular? And these bits of metapsychology that you bring up, isn't their time over?

I shall deal with the last question first, not by addressing its substance, but, *more analitico*[2], by linking it to solitude and to the crisis involving the individual nowadays. *Freudian psychoanalytic metapsychology is, in its entirety, a monument to the ability on the part of the conscious of representing what it will never be able to perceive directly*: the enigma of the body from which the ego itself originates, the enigma of the id, the secrets of the unconscious in the systematic sense of the term. These enigmas and secrets constitute not only a theoretical puzzle; each individual must discover how to recognize this puzzle and how to become acquainted with it within himself, in the terms that best suit him, if he wishes somehow to become a conscious subject. So it is perhaps not a coincidence that the so-called crisis of metapsychology is contemporary to the crisis of the individual in western society.

Let us now return to the two kinds of loneliness—one terrible and the other necessary for the material act of writing—referred to by Freud.

Winnicott's "The Capacity to be Alone" (1958), which instinctively (and therefore preconsciously) comes to mind, began as a paper delivered to the British Society of Psychoanalysis in 1957. In this fine piece of work, Winnicott pursues ways of describing the capacity to be alone from a Freudian and then a Kleinian point of view and then rapidly proceeds from a "three-body" to a "two-body" relationship, which is more congenial to his thinking. The paper is very short but, as often is the case with short works and short dreams, full of implications and meaning. It must be noted that Winnicott accepts the Kleinian hypothesis of an ego that, although immature, already exists at birth: on the basis of this, he argues that "the *ego immaturity is naturally balanced by ego-support* from the mother. In the course of time the individual introjects the ego-supportive mother and in this way becomes able to become alone without frequent reference to the mother or mother symbol" (p. 32). This is based on the assumption, which many disagree with, that the mother "in the early days and weeks, was temporarily identified with her infant, and for the time being *was interested in nothing else* but the care of her own infant" (p. 36; italics added).

This paper could be discussed at length, but what I wish to emphasize here, besides the idea regarding the ego which I have already mentioned, is that (with little comment), Winnicott links his concepts of individuality and of the individual to the capacity for being alone. It is likely that the basis for this can be verified, but only if we restrict the concept of "the capacity to be alone". What does not appear, or is absent from Winnicott's theorizing, in this paper at least, is the notion of a subject. Now it seems to me that individuation and subjectivization are two processes that need to be kept distinct, and that the former is necessary for the latter. But subjectivization is not strictly necessary for daily life and at any rate heavily depends upon the structure of the personal equation that results from overcoming the oedipal conflict and working out the infantile processes during adolescence.

Such a connotation of subject is clearly different and less sophisticated than in Lacan and personally leaves me with the impression that the hidden goal is that of the disappearance of the subject. On the other hand, I believe we can imagine the subject as complex, uneven, lacunal, in continual remaking, but also supported by the functioning of the ego and its conscious areas, which, even if reduced or dramatized, remain nevertheless the sole light guiding us in the darkness of our quest.

In this context, let us once again reflect upon the vicissitudes of writing from the time it is first learned, as well as on the vicissitudes of psychoanalytic writing.

One of the extraordinary things we have a chance to observe about writing is the phenomenon whereby children (whose complex inner world we are acquainted with, thanks, in part, to psychoanalytic research, and whose enormous learning capacity we constantly witness) not only have to make a great effort to learn to write, but are unable to write in the full meaning of the word. Not until adolescence, at the earliest, do children learn how to write, and then only a minority truly become capable of writing. Yet, children are capable of extraordinary thinking.

Cesare Musatti spoke (and also wrote, I believe) of having learnt to write in this sense at around the age of eighteen, when he suddenly understood that he could actually write what he thought and, moreover, could even reflect upon what he had thought by rereading his own writing. Musatti also jokingly maintained that every psychoanalytic congress and every piece of psychoanalytic writing has the same theme: what is psychoanalysis? In that paradoxical style he loved, he thus expressed a truth that we are all acquainted with: psychoanalysis is a totality, and chopping it up into small pieces kills it. But it is a totality because it is a discipline, and a construct, that reflects the unity of the individual and the uniqueness of the subject.

Writing psychoanalysis, from this point of view, is not an impossible undertaking; rather, it is a need that demands to be attended to, a condition of psychic structure. It is also to be understood in the multiple sense, as in the expression "writing one's own psychoanalysis". Each person has his or her own psychoanalytic "theory", and his or her own analytic "history"—a vestige perhaps of the *Familienroman*[3]. Hence the difficulty of our task as editors and readers: we can pretend we are evaluating a text, but we inevitably find ourselves faced with the possibility that the author will not play along, loudly asserting that it was he who was evaluated and not the text.

Paraphrasing a famous saying, we could say that the area *of the page* is the projection of the psychic apparatus' extension. No other derivation is likely. The psyche is extended, but does not know it (Freud, 1941f [1938]).

Thus we find ourselves trapped between two apparently contrasting considerations. On the one hand, it is necessary to write psychoanalysis. On the other hand, writing psychoanalysis is impossible, just as it is impossible to represent, at a conscious level, the uneven, rent, contradictory, and yet unique complexity of the psychic apparatus. And it is likewise impossible to convey psychoanalysis through writing.

Writing in psychoanalysis is therefore concerned with limitations and gaps: limitations of the individual psychic apparatus as well as of the written page and of writing itself, and limitations of logic and reason; notwithstanding distortions and rationalizations, links are effected in order to cover up the discontinuities of the conscious psyche. How rare it is to come across an article that states that a problematic situation has been encountered and then admits that no reasonable solution has been found! How difficult it is to identify a phenomenon and declare at the same time that our eyes are new enough to see it, and our psyches are too old to comprehend it!

The solitude of writing permits a tragic exercise of intellectual honesty that shuns conspiratory solidarity and tolerates a conscious reflection upon oneself, as occurs in another state of consciousness: sleep. It is a narcissistic exercise, an asocial task, that opens up to the social only in wakefulness and in exchanges with readers and colleagues (although it continues to preserve its asocial dimension). Any text that is written only for the sake of writing and not reading is, for me, something analogous to a dream; thus it is often linked to the daydream, as a creation of the compromise that thwarts the realization of material writing.

But this itself becomes a big headache when we are dealing with a task that we term editorial. We certainly cannot enter into the dream, but only evaluate how well a piece approaches social communicability.

It is for this very reason that I believe that, just as consciousness has at its disposal a number of indicators that allow it to identify the contents necessary to undertake its tasks, so the *Rivista*, too, must have a structure that consents to the identification of its material contents. Just as the conscious, by applying a label of origin ("Made in Germany"), identifies the existence of a particular content and establishes, for instance, that it is a dream (i.e. a psychic event concerning something that occurs in sleep), or a memory (i.e. something that can be conceived only by locating it in the past), or a fantasy (i.e. a thought that is not concerned with perception), so the *Rivista* must be able to recognize whether a text falls into the category of pure speculation, or is a description of a remembered state or event (e.g. the recollection of a session), or is something that is in and of itself totally inconceivable but can nevertheless be interpolated for the sake of continuity.

The woe of what we actually do (the meticulous proof-reading, the laying out of a text, the not always felicitous communication with authors, the relations among the editorial group members) takes on a dimension, or a breadth, that should, I believe, be occasionally considered, in order to recognize the utopian scope of this work and reflect with some self-irony on the omnipotent and indispensable illusions that lie behind it.

NOTES

1. *Auffassungen:* concepts.
2. *More analitico:* in analytical fashion.
3. *Familienroman:* family romance.

CHAPTER FIVE

An "ethical code" for authors?

Parthenope Bion Talamo

When I first started thinking about the possibility of producing a paper on writing in psychoanalysis, I had something very simple and practical in mind; not exactly along the lines of an American-style course on "creative writing", but something of that sort. So I was aiming to speak about writing considered as interpersonal communication, which is the area that the people on the board of editors of the *Rivista di Psicoanalisi* usually find themselves dealing with, inasmuch as they function as editors rather than as analysts—and it is also the level on which they find that they have trouble. As I slowly mulled over the (few) ideas that I had on the subject, while being influenced by recent vicissitudes in the Italian Psychoanalytic Society, gradually some thoughts that were connected a little more clearly with the ideal, triangular relationship between the writer, psychoanalysis, and the reader, emerged. At this fatal point (in the sense that chance plays its part, too) Alberto Semi asked me, without the slightest warning, what the title of my paper was going to be . . . and the outcome is something of a hybrid, perhaps rather unpleasant title in fact, even though softened by Alberto's having wisely added a question mark to the original.

In any case, I will try both to keep to my original project and also to blend in with it some of the ideas that came into my mind later, after having tied myself down to a title. The later ideas arose partly in connection with the vicissitudes of the Italian Psychoanalytic Society (I.P.S.), which had undergone a split, and partly from the need to provide the Society with an ethical code to clarify the approach of analysts to the ethics of psychoanalysis. A further train of thought was set in motion through a series of connections that formed in my mind between a few papers, some specifically analytical and others more general, which seemed to me to be pertinent both to the ethical and to the practical side of the question. The first of these, from a chronological point of view, is Jaques' (1981) short paper "The Aims of Psychoanalytical Treatment", which highlights the concept of the "unconscious will to live" (p. 423), describing the behaviour that is a consequence of this will, and how all this lies at the base of our psychoanalytic concept of "normality". The unconscious will to live, as well as linking the single individual to his community through the survival of the species, also becomes an important criterion for the termination of an analysis. It seems to me that with this paper by Jaques at the back of my mind it is possible to perceive that the communication of scientific work between colleagues is vital for the survival of the psychoanalytic community; communication has valences that go beyond the individual's narcissism to become a group link and thus has an extremely important role to play within the group. Most of the papers by analysts that I have looked at tend to deal with the subject of writing mainly, if not exclusively, from the point of view of the writer's inner world; this is certainly an extremely important aspect, but I think that it lies outside the task that I have been set. I will not go into this aspect, then, since it seems to me to be more specifically psychoanalytical and not so necessarily pertinent to the editor's work (I am referring principally to the *Nouvelle Revue de Psychanalyse*, *16*, 1977, and also to the *Revista de Psicoanalisis*, *49* (1), 1993).

To go back to my starting point, that of the usefulness of some sort of guideline to good literary behaviour—not quite a book of etiquette, but getting on that way: I was very much struck by two papers in the first number of *Medifax*. The first of these is by Stephen Lock (1991), the director of the *British Medical Journal*, and the second by Giuseppe Ippolito (1991), who is coordinator of the *Giornale Italiano dell'AIDS*. In this paper, Ippolito indicates standards of behaviour for the referees of scientific papers, showing the need to proceed step by step along a sort of critical path that can be formulated through a series of questions more or less as follows: is the paper original? Is it clearly set out? Does it take the relevant literature into account? Is it complete with bibliography and summary? Is the title appropriate?

These questions which the referee ought to ask himself about every paper that he vets stimulated me to think further about the writing of papers—understood as a moment in which the aim is to communicate something—from the point of view of a psychoanalyst, not restricting myself to simply following this advice as an editor of the *Rivista*. Another *tessera* in the mosaic of my thoughts, placed alongside Ippolito's paper, was the fact that at just about the same time I came across a contract for the publication of a book, in which the author practically has to swear that the text that he presents for publication contains no material that is defamatory or could be offensive, and that the contents are truthful to the best of his knowledge. This contract made me think that publishers and editors must, in fact, really find all sorts of things on their desks . . .

At this point of my meandering around the problem, a colleague very kindly lent me a recent monographic number of the *Revista de Psicoanalisis*, entitled "Escritura in Psicoanalisis", in which one of the papers (Moscone, 1993) presents a whole list of questions—four entire pages of them—which, according to the author, any analyst who wants to embark on the writing of a paper should ask himself. Moscone maintains that the writing of psychoanalysis is essentially different from all other writing and requires a specific procedure; hence the questions, which can be thought of as outlining a sort of "pathway to self-knowledge" for the analyst, covering the ground of the nature of his work with the patients about whom he intends to write, and that of his own attitudes, which can be narcissistic, prejudiced either towards or against a given theory, and so on. It seems to me that Moscone's questions can be a useful complement to Ippolito's more technical ones, although, as we shall see, I do not agree at all with the idea that the writing of psychoanalysis differs substantially from any other scientific writing.

Some of the questions that Moscone poses show a preoccupation with the writer's intellectual honesty, and I think that this problem of honesty, and everything connected with it, is one of the elements that all scientific writing presents (and this is the basic reason why the term "ethical" ended up so uncomfortably in my title). I can agree with Moscone when he states that writing psychoanalysis has a nature of its own, but only insofar as it seems to me that, as we are analysts, we have heuristic tools at our disposal that allow us to enquire into our "doing" in a new and much more powerful way than was possible earlier (or is possible even now if we restrict ourselves to the use of exegesis and hermeneutics, which Moscone quotes as being inadequate). However, this does not prevent the useful exportation to other fields of the results of a psychoanalytically informed enquiry into writing. This persuasion of mine also implies the idea that, fundamentally, scientific method is one, and that it can be studied apart from the specific contents of the single sciences. I hold, furthermore, that the study of scientific method, which includes the communication of scientific activity both to colleagues and to society at large, cannot do without a psychoanalytical enquiry that clarifies the ways in which both scientific method and communication are structured. I intend to discuss this second aspect now, and it seems to me that it is possible to embark on a specifically psychoanalytically informed enquiry, with the aim of attaining something useful and practical, even though what I am going to say at this point may look like a long digression.

Which are the pertinent psychoanalytical theories? Although it may seem anti-historical, I am led by the nature of my argument to start with Bion and go on to Freud—a "minor" Freud, but most significant for the intuitions expressed.

In *Learning from Experience*, Bion (1962b) speaks of the way in which the individual's relationships with his inner and his external objects—with the whole world—are carried on under the aegis of particular mental states that emotionally colour both the links that are set up and the very setting up of the links themselves. Bion chooses three specific, more or less hegemonic, states—Love, Hate, and Knowledge, indicated by the letters L, H, and K. He also speaks of the three complementary states, –L, –H, and –K, in which the positive characteristic of moving towards an object, to enrich both it and the subject, becomes instead a "draining away" from the object, a "depriving" it of the quality in question. In our context, we could say that a scientific paper written under the aegis of K is one whose content has been adequately worked through in the author's mind, and that the latter can feel that he has a reasonably good command of the ideas he has expressed, which also comes from having sufficient experience and maturation, from a sufficiently long study of his particular subject. A paper, on the other hand, that has been written under the aegis of –K, since –K is not simply the opposite of K, not only does not have these characteristics but is written—is thought—in such a way as not to give any new information to the reader, and does not stimulate the latter to produce new thoughts for himself. Writing of this sort is in no way interactive with the reader, it does not allow a dialogue with him, it is almost as though it were dead. I expect that we can all call to mind an example of this sort of writing; for me, at the top of the series (or perhaps the nadir), is a history of the birth of the State of Israel, which is also a biography of Theodor Herzl (Elon, 1975). This is a book that, most unusually for me, I have never been able to finish, because it made me feel that it was never going to get off the ground. It seemed to me that it was a sort of hagiography that went on repeating *ad nauseam* that Herzl was a brilliant man who had had a brilliant idea, without ever going into the details of what he had thought or how his ideas had developed. (Obviously, this is not an analytical book but has pretensions in the direction of scientific historiography; I realize that my reaction to the text might merely be idiosyncratic, but even when I take it up again, years after the first attempt, it has the same frustrating effect on me. Among the books at the other end of the scale, one would certainly place Freud's works.)

It would also be possible to write a scientific paper under the aegis of L; in fact, I am sure that a good scientific paper, well written and which thrills the reader with enthusiasm, cannot be without feelings of love for psychoanalysis, for the creative act of writing, for the use of the tongue in which it is written and the appropriate language, and feelings of love too towards those people, as yet unknown, who will read the paper. (Naturally, the person who was best able to express this concept could not but be a poet, who consigns the beauty of his loved one to posterity in order to keep it alive, and in so doing implies gratitude towards those who will, by reading, further his project: ". . . So long as men can breathe and eyes can see, / So long lives this, and this gives life to thee.") Again, a paper written under the aegis of −L, always supposing that it is possible to write in such a colourless mental state of indifference and emptiness, would be extremely difficult to tolerate. Perhaps the chapter of *The Interpretation of Dreams* (Freud, 1900a) that Freud found so difficult to write, the one in which he "had" to review the previous literature on the subject, might be considered an example of writing in which one catches just the faintest whiff of −L (Jones, 1953, I: p. 358).

We can draw up the hypothesis, then, that a good piece of scientific writing has the characteristics of L and K links. But does this hypothesis lead us anywhere? It takes us in two directions, I think: in the first place, a paper written exclusively as a form of knowledge, that is, under the aegis of K, might well remain a private fact, without the third pole—the reader, the public—being called into the question. When the L link comes into the picture, this third pole becomes more important, because love for psychoanalysis and for writing requires that there be someone to receive the communication, in the same way in which a musician is not complete if there is never anyone to listen to him.

Calling the reader into the question, however, sets off other psychological mechanisms, which, as far as I know, have not been much studied with reference to groups. I am referring in particular to projective identification (on the writer's part) and to the capacity for toleration, on the part of the group of readers (or listeners, if the paper is read at a conference) (Bion, 1962a), acting as a container for the projective identifications. (In the case of a conference, the interplay of projective identifications, in both directions, is much more evident and can lead to modification of the paper even while it is being read.) All of us may—and do—have conscious expectations about the way in which our mental products will be received, whether they be in the form of a conference, a seminar, or a publication for reading in private, which range from the Nobel Prize, or the "Booker", the "Strega", or the "Goncourt", at one end of the scale, to bad eggs and tomatoes, or the exclusion from civil society for the rest of one's days, at the other. In some way or other we usually manage to deal with these fantasies so that they do not interfere too outrageously with our capacity for work.

I am less optimistic, however, as far as our capacity for dealing with projective identifications is concerned, particularly the less realistic ones (which can in some ways be likened to unconscious expectations). When I mentioned mental products a little way back, the idea of a very small baby also came into my mind, depositing its faeces in its mother's lap. How many of the papers that have been sent to the *Rivista* have been unconsciously accompanied by messages that would have been appropriate *x* years previously, when he, the author, was held in his mother's arms? How many papers seem to need maternal care to clean and tidy them up, and how many have been felt—correctly, I think—as hostile and arrogant attacks on the reader? In how many papers does one come across howlers that make one think that the author must have had strong feelings of envy, hatred, or who knows what—perhaps simply deathly boredom—towards the author or authors whom he is himself quoting? As an example of this sort of thing, I would like to quote a well-known and esteemed psychoanalyst who, in a paper that seems to have been produced for teaching purposes, states:

> . . . the first group considers that the aim of interpretative work is to produce a deep understanding, which will allow the patient to carry out his wishes without anxiety or feelings of guilt; the others (for example Bion, 1976) say that analysis aims at reaching a state "free from remembering, desiring or understanding".

("The first group", in this passage, consists of Anna Freud, Eissler, Fenichel, Greenson, Lampl-de Groot, Loewenstein, Neyraut, Sandler, Zetzel; while "the others", apart from Bion includes Balint, Bouvet, Giovacchini, Kernberg, Khan, M. Klein, Little, Rosenfeld, Segal, Winnicott—two rather mixed bags, though united in the author's mind, it would seem, by a certain amount of spleen—Cremerius, 1985, p. 115.)

If it is to be supposed that some of these meta-messages that show through between the lines of scientific papers are in fact signs pointing to the presence of projective identifications, it is also true that the person who is reading has to come to terms with his own reactions as "container"; he has to decide, that is, whether the acidic comment or the excited enthusiasm that rises unexpectedly to consciousness are really in tune with the work they are reading, or whether there is not something excessive in these reactions, which might be a way of responding to a projective identification that is felt to be hampering the course of thought and yet needs to be taken in and seen to. I think that some of our difficulties as readers (and as writers) may lie on deep levels of the unconscious where there is in fact an interplay of projective identifications that imply an incorrect, since unrealistic, attribution of characteristics and functions.

One of the problems that we meet if we try not only to ferret out this sort of difficulty but also to act in order to resolve it to a certain extent is our (correct) sense of reserve over using psychoanalytical concepts, theories, and understandings outside the analytical context proper. But we go on being analysts, that is to say, people whose sensitivity towards certain types of behaviour should be sharpened by the work we do, and this sort of sensitivity cannot simply be turned off outside the consultation-room. This means that sometimes we find that we are faced with a scientific paper that disturbs us, maybe violently, and that furthermore we have to face up to these feelings and also interact in the outside world, in our dealings with the colleague who has written the paper. So far, the structure of the *Rivista* has involved "blind" reading, which can be a help, in the sense of allowing a freer expression of one's unease, but there comes a moment when one of us has to get into touch with the author and say something to him, preferably in a civil fashion, to give him support, if necessary, and at the same time do this without being intrusive.

At this point, we can turn to the other branch that stems off from the hypothesis of a paper written under the aegis of L and K (I am not taking into consideration works written under the aegis of H, though I think that they exist). The writing of a scientific paper entails not only the creation of links, internal ones in the first place, with the subject of the paper, but also—at a stage that is either earlier or contemporary with the creation of inner links—many passages from the paranoid–schizoid position to the depressive one and vice versa. It seems to me that usually this is anything but pleasant, being accompanied by feelings of anxiety and a general sense of malaise, of which the well-known block when confronted with the white page (or equivalent) is just one example. It is an unpleasant situation—principally, I think, because these processes are deeply unconscious during most of our waking life, and having to perceive them consciously, even if only very dimly, undoubtedly entails the arousal of anxiety and feelings of pain and loss. Freud was aware of this sort of problem, as we can see from his note on the prehistory of psychoanalytic technique, in which, *à propos* of free association, he talks about creative writing and mentions the article by Ludwig Börne, "The Art of Becoming an Original Writer in Three Days" (Freud, 1920b). Börne says that one must write notes for three days on everything that comes into one's head, as a method for becoming a writer; he then remarks that in reality the individual lacks moral courage, not ideas. Here it seems that Freud almost prepares the ground for the much later theory of the paranoid--schizoid position (and the oscillations between this and the depressive position) as a constitutive element of creative thought, but the comment on the "moral qualities" of the writer is also pertinent to my idea, though it is still vague and not clearly formulated, that writing psychoanalysis also calls an ethical element into the field.

At this point, my original intention of writing an "ethical code" for the authors of psychoanalytical texts seems to have disappeared completely, and to be rather difficult to retrieve, after this long theoretical digression, mainly on a limited aspect of Bion's theory of thinking. But there is in fact a connection, and perhaps more than one, between two subjects that appear so far apart.

If we now take a look at a series of "defects" in writing (many of which can probably be found in this paper I am writing/reading), perhaps we can form a few ideas about the way they come into being and hence suggest a system for limiting them—a system that will in fact be akin to an "ethical code" . This kinship exists, to my mind, because those aspects of a written text that simply appear under the guise of technical "defects", so to say, are in reality the expression of subterranean states of psychological malaise of various sorts. An ethical code for the psychoanalyst/writer of scientific papers could then be useful to the author, as a sort of memorandum that would allow him to check—through the external signs that he comes across in the way the text is written—the state of health of his own creativity, of his relationship with his work, and of his relationships with his colleagues. This sort of code can be considered to be "ethical" insofar as our working tool, our mind, "must" be kept in good working order; it is part of the duties one takes on if one decides to become a psychoanalyst, duties that concern not only our relationships with our patients or our colleagues, but also those that we have towards ourselves. (In the same way in which someone who wants to be a musician or a neurosurgeon, for example, has to give up those sports that strain the hands excessively, we have to keep an eye on the efficiency of our mental functioning and protect it.)

The first "technical defects" that come to my mind are the following:

1. the use of a language that is too specific, verging on jargon for those in the know, in the context of psychoanalytical theorization, which cannot reasonably be held to be of common use and hence known to everyone (I am thinking of Winnicott-talk, Bion-talk, and so on);
2. the use of terms in foreign languages without an explicatory note, where a term in the language used for the rest of the text could be adopted or, failing this, an adequate explanation of the foreign term;
3. the lack of a summary;
4. the lack of a bibliography;
5. the use of clinical vignettes that do not seem to be connected to the theoretical part or do not illustrate it adequately;
6. a confused and untidy presentation of the contents, which gives the impression of thoughts jumping here and there;
7. the quotation of a mass of bibliographical data that suffocate rather than illuminate the author's thesis;
8. the use of justifications for the correctness and validity of a theory made exclusively with reference to other theories instead of on the basis of clinical experience:

"Freud says . . . " is not enough to guarantee the truth of an author's statement about a theory of his own.

It seems to me that the first group of defects, from 1 to 4, has a ground in fantasies in which the readers are invested with various sorts of parental characteristics. The use of (1) jargon and of (2) untranslated terms in other languages has a great deal to do with fantasies of infantile omnipotence; while the lack of (3) summary and of (4) bibliography seems, rather, to be connected with fantasies that consider potential readers as "containers" that "must" busy themselves with cleaning up and with completing the things that the child has left undone.

The defects that I have gathered together under points (5) and (6)—inappropriate use of clinical illustrations and a confused and untidy presentation—would seem, rather, to stem from a sort of stickiness, as though the author had got rather mixed up in the paranoid-schizoid position and were not quite able to free himself from it to make that last passage to the depressive position, which would allow a better tidying up of the whole paper.

The last two defects—(7) too many bibliographical data and and (8) validation "between theories"—concern the fantasy relationships between the writer and the group that is his reference point in the real world. In our case, this is the I.P.S., certainly, but also "Psychoanalysis" and furthermore "*La Rivista*", which is often felt to be a sort of bugbear among those who do not have much to do with it. (Even I, who ought to feel that I "belong" to the *Rivista* and who should have felt that I was playing on home ground during the day-long study-group, found that I had a good many qualms, in the first place while writing this paper, and in the second while presenting it.) The unconscious fantasies at the base of this sort of situation are rather paranoid, the interlocutor *Rivista* being felt to represent something imposing that requires a rigidly orthodox attitude on the part of the postulant, without which it will not be possible to placate it. The nature of this orthodoxy is not defined in the fantasy, and the minor sort of orthodoxy that is actually required of the authors, outlined in the "Notes for Authors"—for many years defined as "Standards"—is happily ignored most of the time, perhaps because it is of no use for quieting the unconscious fantasies?

This grouping of the most frequently met defects also corresponds to different areas of problems, which range from the relationship with oneself, to the one with our discipline, and with our colleagues, and all three of these areas can be suffused with feelings of love or knowledge to a greater or lesser degree. The ideal situation, a sort of "state of grace" for the writer of psychoanalysis, would correspond to one in which he feels that he has a tranquil mastery of the subject, he knows that he will not damage the patients of whom he wishes to speak, he wishes to present his ideas to colleagues towards whom he has friendly feelings, and from whom he expects to receive a respectful hearing that might give rise to reasoned criticism from which he thinks that he will be able to learn something. Briefly, he expects both to give and to receive through the act of communication that he is about to undertake. (It was pointed out to me during the debate that this does not correspond to an ideal state but rather to an idealized one. This is a valid criticism, and I am bringing it in here not only because of its intrinsic value, but also because it throws light on the way in which both my conscious and unconscious preoccupation with very uneasy feelings connected with the current splitting tendencies in the I.P.S. can colour the formulation of a theory, in an idealizing way in this case, letting fall by the wayside those aspects of healthy aggressiveness that are also part of the humus from which a new idea is born. This aggressiveness is recognized as such and at times arouses polemical reactions in the listeners or readers.)

We have now reached the fateful question: What sort of an ethical code, then, and how is it to be drawn up? Given the precedents of Ippolito and Moscone, it seems that it will necessarily have to be a questionnaire, an enquiry, not the Tables of the Law.

But if, as I think, this sort of ethical code ought basically to be part of one's own self-analysis, how can one draw up a set of questions that will be valid for everyone? Semi's famous question mark turns out to be an important integration of my title, not just something that softens its harshness. Writing psychoanalysis, communicating with our colleagues, is an integral part of the scientific side of our work, and the latter cannot be separated from a continual questioning of oneself on the meaning of what one is doing. Perhaps the most important part of the analyst's thinking in the here and now of the session comes about through his formulation of those specific questions that are valid in that moment in order to push his thoughts still further, though most of the time, of course, he keeps these questions to himself, does not express them out loud, and does not inflict them on the patient. Therefore each of us might amuse himself by drawing up his own personal ethical code, changing the questions in it from time to time, according to his evolution, trying to be as honestly aware as is possible of his own emotions and unconscious tendencies.

But it is by no means easy to carry out self-analysis—this is the reason why our patients allow us to work—and perhaps it would be a good idea to have a friend to whom one could entrust a reading of the manuscript *in fieri*[1]—someone who, without going into details intended to reveal the writer's unconscious, could say to him: "Look, here you sound a bit fed up, here it's not so clear—and if you changed the order of those two paragraphs? . . ." This is not the role of the editors of a psychoanalytic journal, although sometimes I get the feeling that it is what the aspiring authors propose we should do. Perhaps one of the problems that we ought to face up to as members of an editorial board is precisely that of a sort of "bringing up" of our authors, with a greater awareness than we have had so far as to what is involved. We can gain this both from technical hints like those in Ippolito's paper and from our professional awareness of the unconscious aspects of writing and communicating.

NOTE

1. *In fieri:* in preparation.

CHAPTER SIX

Experiences and considerations of a "reader" of psychoanalysis

Fausto Petrella

The foremost purpose of a meeting between the individuals concerned with the publication of a psychoanalytic journal—the editors and the "readers"—should, in my view, be an eminently practical one. The aim is not to investigate the role of psychoanalytic writing in the emotional life and fantasy of the psychoanalyst, perhaps by invoking Derrida. Nor is it to discuss and formulate a standard of scientific rigour for psychoanalysis, with an appeal to some updated thesis of epistemology. My intention is to have an open discussion about our experience as "readers"—that is, individuals who have agreed to perform an anonymous, largely unrecognized task on a text written by an equally anonymous author. When I speak of the "reader", it is to this figure that I refer and not to the imaginary addressee of the text or to any particular living reader. My starting point will be the specific experience of this reader, who must formulate and express an opinion, and whose tasks are at once well- and ill-defined. This should give a pragmatic orientation to what I have to say. The overall aim should be one of improvement. But in which direction? One might be that of defining this function, determining the existence and efficacy of generally acceptable evaluative instruments and criteria, clarifying the way evaluations concerning each contribution evolve, and making explicit the characteristics and limits of such evaluations. The goal, then, is to arrive, if not at a relative homogeneity, at least at a certain transparency in the reader's operations, thereby promoting competence and mutual trust. This does not mean that we should strive for an impossible harmonization or a monotonous unison: what is needed is not so much a set of commonly agreed-upon criteria as an occasion to meet and discuss the criteria that are already being employed. The reader's function, if not privileged, is certainly specific and allows a few observations from a particular perspective. It is this specificity and the way it is made use of by both the readers and the editors that concerns me here. To do this, it will be necessary to set aside our mutual anonymity and to share experiences.

It may be useful to return to the *past* for a moment.

The board of readers was originally proposed in accordance with the habitual practice of scientific journals with claims to seriousness of having a committee of anonymous referees who are distinct from the management and from the editorial board and who are asked to express themselves in writing about the characteristics and publishability of each paper. This function—the fact that it was considered necessary for the *Rivista*—was in itself a mark of the great changes that have taken place over the years in the Italian Psychoanalytic Society. It was no accident that an innovative proposal of this nature was strongly supported by several so-called younger colleagues, if I remember correctly. In other words, the need was felt for a change from the family-style, oligarchical management of psychoanalytic matters to the government of a much vaster community that expressed theoretical and clinical positions both quite heterogeneous in content and varied in form. The *Rivista*, being the official scientific organ of the Italian Psychoanalytic Society, reflected this change faithfully and in a certain sense highlighted and intensified it. The number of analysts had been growing over the years, and therefore, although the papers submitted for publication were not multiplying at the same rate, it became increasingly important to provide some form of responsible appraisal and "imprimatur". It should be remembered that the *Rivista di Psicoanalisi* is a strictly societal organ, reserved for members of the Italian Psychoanalytic Society and for occasional foreign guests belonging to the International Psychoanalytic Association. The work of non-psychoanalysts and students is generally not published. The principal purchasers of the journal are analysts themselves—they are, that is, those interested in research and in the study of our field—a category that all of us, and not least the publisher, hope is numerous and qualified.

Let us now consider the group dynamics that a journal like ours necessarily implies, connected with what is called psychoanalytic thought and with scientific production. It is not my intention to propose a thorough analysis of this complex situation but only to point out the existence of a series of problems of obvious importance.

Scientific journals, more than books, are an agile medium for the circulation of ideas and the communication of information on the state of research. They attest to the competence and skill of the authors. They corroborate current paradigms and indicate possibilities for their use. On occasion they break with the paradigms of mainstream science, for which the journal serves as a forum of the written word and the congress as a stage for live performance. But in addition to these functions there are others that concern the group's relationship with itself and with what is external to it as well as the relationship of each author with his colleagues and with the discipline. At periodic intervals the *Rivista*, unlike a book, allows the variegated and pluralistic experience of everyday clinical work—fragmentary, on the edge of suffering, ephemeral in its fleetingness, typically personal and idiosyncratic—to leave the subjective dimension of solitary reflection. Experience and practice plunge into writing, thirst for a place in the lexicon, strive for consensus and to be lifted up into the skies of theory, or in any case to be granted some form of eternalness, by becoming part of group culture and of the community.

A journal, ours or any other of the same kind, may initially be part of the foundations of a group—a component, that is, of a society or association. Subsequently, however, it must reflect and reconfirm the group's identity over time and constitute what is called a tradition. In other words, it must continually represent, despite on-going changes, the same picture, a sort of family portrait of itself and of a handful of ancestors. This kind of common ground, grounded in the reassurance deriving from shared knowledge, has become increasingly problematic and hazy as the number of members has grown and as the generations have passed. If the family becomes overextended, it becomes more and more difficult to recognize oneself in this enlarged picture, and the feeling of a common identity—that of the community of psychoanalysts—becomes more faint and uncertain. One begins to lose hold of this grounding in genealogy, filiation, and affiliation, in which the ancestors and a shared analytic experience guarantee membership in the community and even in a broader international movement. It becomes necessary to turn to the world of thoughts and ideas: a vaster and more open-ended superindividual reality, which is farther from specific founding personalities and much closer to concreteness, to ideas, conceptions, and applications. It is this reality, made up of experiences and language, that must be the object of publication and collective circulation.

The creation of a committee of readers is part of an operation designed to "normalize" the *Rivista di Psicoanalisi* and adapt it to certain standards of the culture of science-in-journals and to the constraints this science imposes on its practitioners: limitations on text length, precise rules of uniformity for references and quotes, and a whole range of conventions concerning layout and graphics. A certain number of formal limitations does not hurt. After all, the rules imposed on sonnet writers did not prevent the creation of great and even marvellous communicative events despite the rigid confines of a hypercodified poetic form. What is more, limitations on length, for example, are underpinned by an idea of democracy and discipline: everyone, or very many, who accept these constraints may take the floor.

The task of the reader, who works to no personal advantage as he exercises his own dispassionate (but also passionate) judgement on the most qualifying aspect of analytic work, provoked in me a series of different reactions. Initially, these reactions were negative.

To begin with, this task was made extremely arduous by the rather unsettling, chaotic disunity of theoretical perspectives and approaches. I also remember quite well how I first reacted to the prescribed anonymity. There were fewer analysts then than today, and those who wrote were a minority within the minority.

I found the anonymity of the reader and author an unpleasant and pointless hypocrisy: Who couldn't recognize the author, especially if, as was often the case, he cited his own work in the references? Wouldn't it have been possible to take an anonymous jab at the author, pretending not to know him? It seemed that in this way we were institutionalizing the bad habit of "throwing the stone and hiding the hand". Or the error could be aggravated by penalizing a respected author by mistaking him for a faltering beginner. Considering that all analysts are always to some extent beginners, it was an easy trap to fall into. But what made me most uneasy was that my idealized image of the analytic community, which I associated with frankness and the possibility of open polemics, seemed to vacillate. On more than one occasion I sent in my little reader's reports proudly signed, since it seemed absurd, and even unacceptable, that one should not assume the responsibility for one's own judgement, especially concerning recognizable authors. But I was rather naively underestimating both the socially positive role of hypocrisy and the advantage of this "double blind" for the editors and directors. These individuals, in fact, maintained their sovereignty of judgement concerning both the anonymous experts and the authors (who in the end were not at all anonymous for those who had the last word). Clearly, this two- or even threefold blindness—a myth with oedipal, or rather anti-oedipal overtones, since castration is ritually anticipated—serves to reduce the level of conflict between author and editor and to reinforce, but at the same time to dilute, the responsibility for a possible rejection, with everything that such a rejection may mean for the author . . . All this seemed to aim at the constitution of a scientific body cleansed of potentially deadly tensions, thus leaving room for an inextricable mix comprising the defence of doctrinal purity, the genealogy of the author and the group, and the institutionalization of scientific and cultural power. On the other hand, those who feel a certain nostalgia for those fascinating and at times brutal exchanges of opinion between editor and master concerning authors and articles, of the type that we find occasionally in the correspondence between Jung (editor of the *Jahrbuch*) and Freud, should also bear in mind the trajectory, and the outcome, of that relationship. But let us not further complicate the already complicated matter of today with references to the archaeology of our field.

A review like ours, which we might call a statutory and non-partisan organ, has first and foremost certain obvious, modest *documentary functions*. It *must* publish articles that, aside from their specific value, bear witness to what is being thought or done. It is here that one should be able to discover what psychoanalysts think, what their practice and theory is about, how they conceive of their work. It is obvious, then, that the *Rivista* must offer space for, as it were, the convergence of divergences and allow for the juxtaposition, the concentration and comparison, the contrast and mirroring of radically different positions. Provided that they are psychoanalytic positions—which cannot be assured *ipso facto* by the author's membership in the circle of analysts, even though a non-institutional definition of what psychoanalytic means could raise numerous problems.

I was less reluctant to accept the anonymity of the role of reader when I realized that despite my efforts to unmask their identity, it was increasingly common that authors remained anonymous: trying to discover the identity of an author is a very instructive game, but too often it is very difficult or even impossible to win. Once I was forced to examine without guidance the merits and contents of the articles, I became immediately aware of the need for considerable tolerance and openness towards the most disparate ideas and positions. In the end, the documentary role of the review rendered the job of evaluating the publishability of a work less burdensome than expected; and in any case, as it turned out, I have never seen an article about which I had expressed a substantially negative opinion go unpublished. Eventually I understood that the reader has a merely advisory function, while the final judgement is reserved for the readers' readers—that is, the editorial board and editor-in-chief of the review, both of whom may judge on the basis of criteria that are in conflict with the opinion of anonymous readers. The point is not secondary, because this makes it impossible to call the reader a "referee", a reviewer whose opinion is significantly more binding than that of a "reader".

The reader, then, did not have the power to decide the life and death of a creature presented to the temple, nor even to determine whether a paper was good or excellent, as opposed to mediocre or bad. In this way the function of the reader came to be one of collaboration, aimed at improving the product by offering a critical and, in the final analysis, therapeutic contribution: a contribution to the care of the text, to use a meaningful expression bordering both on the medical and on the maternal. The changes effected were often not merely cosmetic but truly delicate operations that raised questions about the very content of the text.

A text that presents itself in society should be clean-shaven and, if not elegantly dressed, at least orderly and appropriate in appearance. Casual clothes are permitted, but they should not be the fruit of negligence or naiveté in writing and, ultimately, in thought. Looks count in writing as well. Form and content pursue each other, and I do not think that I can be accused of excessive aestheticism for saying so. The reader is certainly required to be tolerant of positions different from his own, but this tolerance must not turn into an excessive suspension of judgement, refusing to navigate between the crags of the debatable. But then what and how are we to judge, if we must respect the orientations of authors with whom we do not at all agree? Even from the perspective of this prudent respect there are many things that can be judged and debated about a psychoanalytic paper. I will list a few of the elements that I feel should be taken into account:

- the relationships between the conjectures brought to bear, the argumentative apparatus, and the descriptive aspects of the materials presented; even the proportions between these ingredients can determine the quality of the dish;
- whether, and to what extent, the attention the author draws to method and technique is reflected in his argumentation;
- the balance between mimesis, diegesis, and comment in the clinical account; how well the author controls the oscillation between metaphor and conceptualization in his overall presentation;
- the awareness of ideological aspects, of the options and criteria employed at each theoretical and clinical level, and the way in which all this is presented and is transformed into expository discourse.

There is not one of the aspects mentioned above that does not have a decisive impact on the evaluation of the quality of a piece of psychoanalytic writing, and in my experience as a reader I have often been struck by the discordant and curious effects of the author's insufficient or poor control over them. Below I have listed in note form some typical examples of commonplaces that can compromise the quality of a paper:

- a certain disdain for metapsychology and its arbitrariness, while at the same employing its concepts and unilaterally introducing new, no less arbitrary options
- the criticism of Freud and of certain aspects of his approach while drawing on arguments found in Freud himself, apparently unknown to the author; the same may hold true of the criticism of other authors
- the introduction of new paradigms or simply of new terms without considering that these may enter into contradiction with other and different assumptions of the discourse and method employed in the text
- the uncontrolled proliferation of analogies, allusions to myth, and clinical rituals, in the form, for example, of sketches that claim to give an empirical foundation to the argument but instead often create more problems than clarity
- the disproportionate, or even irrelevant, interacting with or embarking on lofty cultural issues (aesthetics, ethics, logic, etc.), for which the psychoanalyst is not particularly well equipped and which must be approached with caution and rigour in order to be treated fruitfully for psychoanalysis
- the adoption of philosophical and literary technical jargon to substitute the language of psychoanalysis, with the typical result that it is often difficult to distinguish the enrichment deriving from such operations from adulteration and abuse
- a tendency to advance metaphysical assertions and options that allegedly arise from the materials and experience of the analysis, but which seem to reflect, rather, the author's "scarce awareness that one is interpreting", as is said of certain responses to the Rorschach test
- the straying of the theoretical and clinical discourse which ultimately leads to an imbalance in the text; this may be due to excessive references to other disciplines (from mathemat-

ics to logic, from narratology to epistemology) or to an uncontrolled proliferation of metaphors, though metaphoric discourse is admittedly unavoidable

- the belief that a useful remedy for all this consists in turning either to clinical material (the case history, the "sketch", the suffered exposition of one's countertransference) or to some theoretical discovery considered to be decisive.

Having pointed out these sins, which are only a few of the most common, I will not be the one to cast the first or the second stone. Nor do I believe it possible to prescribe true remedies—by preaching continence, for example. What I can propose are not remedies but simply suggestions, such as the appeal to temperance, the rule of Occam's razor (the fundamental methodological principle that prescribes that the formulation of all scientific theories should follow the famous maxim: *Entia non sunt multiplicanda praeter necessitatem*[1]), an invitation to a sense of proportion—proportion and congruence between theory and the clinical; between analogies, metaphors, and illustrations on the one hand and concepts on the other; between description, delineations of the workings of the psychic apparatus, and argumentation; between efforts to persuade and the presentation of proof. It is impossible to prescribe, or perhaps even recommend, a precise balance among all these elements. This much is obvious. The awareness of the conjectural character of many psychoanalytic propositions, the control over form, the "play" between, on the one hand, the flexibility of the author's associations and correlations and, on the other, the precision of his writing; these are all factors that have to do both with the scientific quality of a text and with what is generally attributed to its *style*. We know that style is in part rooted in the author's personal fantasy and that this fantasy induces the sort of reflection that flows headlong onto the written page, even to the point of becoming identical with it.

But writing is also a place in which the author's megalomania, great and small, expresses itself. This megalomania is often legitimate, just as it may be legitimate to express polemics, impatience, and many other feelings that outside the written page would be damaging and blameworthy. Artistic prose—that is, stylistically controlled writing—and scientific prose converge in an original way in the construction of the scientific discourse of psychoanalysis, and they are to some extent both necessary, as we have learned from the texts of Freud. Ideally, science strives for a form of truth that exhibits its own proof, confirmation, and reproducibility. All these things are possible in our case, but they are condemned to remain only *experimentum mentis* and have an insurmountable element of uncertainty. On the basis of all this, it is evident that if the reader were really to embark on extremely precise appraisals, his task would be extraordinarily complex. In any case, the reader's judgement should not be too personal, nor should he be overly influenced by his own "vision" of the treatment and the analysis. Personally, I have always tried to go beyond this direct comparison and to identify points of analytic interest at a more general level, which may serve as parameters for judging the quality and publishability of a paper.

Certainly, not only the reader but also the author who writes for the *Rivista* should know to what and to whom the review is addressed. If it is to circulate among specialists or followers of a particular school, a certain exotericism—in vocabulary, style, and subject matter—may be justifiable. To the initiates it would not even appear to be esoteric, since they would understand each other even in obscurity, and the obscure discourse would confirm their status as initiates. But there also is a responsibility towards the "outsider", towards the reader who is not a member of the system but who can contribute to the configuration of the ideal addressee of the *Rivista* and of its articles. Personally, when I write, I always keep in mind the non-specialist. Ideally—and *si licet parva* and so forth . . . in other words, if I may be permitted—the same paper can be designed to be read at different levels, as great art teaches us. As for non-specialists, some might become irritated at not understanding very much, others might be dazzled by the obscurity, and we might find, as in fact we do, the most varied positions towards all this. It would always be possible for someone to unmask the emptiness that lies behind the layer of textual tinsel and remind us that the emperor is naked. This *enfant terrible*, sworn enemy of textual theatrics, could at this point consider his critical task accomplished. On the other hand, he might—once the emperor is dead—propose something else, of his own, for example. In this way the game goes on, the infinite entertainment of writing and criticizing. But, aside from the game, at issue are decisive aspects of the credibility of psychoanalysis and its therapeutic practice, and more simply the vitality and appeal of a review should reflect the state of health of a scientific society.

I do not believe that all these problems can be solved by listing a series of criteria to be followed. This could be done, but I think that they are obvious enough to everyone. Who wouldn't agree that a piece of psychoanalytic writing should be characterized by sobriety and clarity and that each paper should state its aim, begin with some thesis—clinical or theoretical—that should, at the conclusion, be, if not proven, at least examined thoroughly or clarified? All of us feel that one should always respect not only the grammar and the syntax of the language but also the vocabulary of our discipline and of those brought to bear in any given study. We all agree that one should avoid the abuse of neologisms, which is rarely justified, and jargon. (I had occasion recently to hear a colleague read a paper at a psychoanalytic conference and justify the obscurity of his language with the need—the reasons for which were not stated—to reinvent the terminology of psychoanalysis in a personal way. His neologisms, he said, would require a key for their interpretation, best dealt with in footnotes, which, however, would be inappropriate at a conference!)

I have sometimes thought, on reading certain papers, that "here we could use some plain common sense". But we all know that "common sense" alone would never have given us psychoanalysis and that it is the task of writing to contain the boldness of thought and of unbridled theoretical fantasy, rendering them effective by the demands of argumentation, style, and conceptual elaboration.

Finally, I would add that the reader should take an active part in the present (re-)definition of the *Rivista's* aims and of his mandate to evaluate papers. Whatever this mandate might be, certain fundamental criteria must be observed, such as attention to form, to the connection between form and content, and to the proportion between thesis and proof.

Psychoanalytic writing has a great variety of "subgenres", which should be identified and measured against the general characteristics that we are striving for in the *Rivista*. Two of these are the *clinical paper* and the *theoretical paper*. But we also have the *clinical–theoretical* genre and the *theoretical–clinical* one. Since these are circular genres, rotating on their own axes, it is necessary, as at the roulette, to observe where the author's "ball" comes to rest and to make sure that there are no tricks that tilt the game wheel and its truth.

There are also *centripetal papers*, which keep coming back to psychoanalysis, though taking more or less extravagant detours to other sciences. From mathematics to psychology, there is no field that cannot be integrated into our peculiar discipline, including astronomy, ecology, optics, the arts, alchemy, immunology, chemistry . . . And then there are *centrifugal papers*, which drift more or less visibly until, abandoning both clinic and theory, they weigh anchor to sail to new waters. As we have no accurate territorial map, it may be difficult to determine when one has deviated from the legitimate routes of psychoanalysis. Indeed, even Freud might find that some of his writings would be rejected by a contemporary committee of readers.

It is not uncommon to come across *"gut" papers* in which the author feels that to be up-to-date he must exhibit his own emotions, his *entrailles*, and those of his patient. Generally, we find negative, depressive feelings or feelings of laceration and anxiety (due to separations, mournings, the loss of various things, . . .). The stylistic range of these outpourings is quite varied but certainly not sufficient to qualify a paper as psychoanalytic, although it constitutes an essential aspect of our work that can hardly be ignored. Those who choose to ignore this aspect risk falling into the unhappy genre of the *intellectual* or *intellectualistic paper;* these texts are alienated from feelings, and both patient and analyst are merely a bothersome means to scientific illumination, a necessary obstacle in the path of a cognitive construction. "Gut" papers are generally classified as "clinical" and intellectual articles as "theoretical".

Not infrequently, we find *polemical writing*: polemics against some aspect of technique, against a certain concept of therapy, or against some theoretical position. On occasion such papers are clothed in a more or less effective humorous or sarcastic veil. Of course, Polemos is one of the great divine patrons of writing, and personally I do not believe I have ever written anything that did not contain some conscious or subtle attack against someone, at times so well concealed that only a few intimates would notice, but at times quite explicit. In company, however, polemics should not be exaggerated and pushed across the threshold of *bon ton*: no one can raise his voice in your living room without becoming unpleasant after a while. A muffled tone is generally more appreciated and produces effects of reassuring equilibrium. Monotony is preferable to wild shrieking.

Naturally, boring papers do not make up a genre apart. But they often appear in a rather well-defined genre, which we might call *normal papers*. Normal papers have the principal aim of corroborating the stability of psychoanalytic discourse, its conformity with some accepted and recognizable aspect of culture, and of showing that the author is in line with those aspects. This genre often has precise textual markers and presents specific lexical and expository options.

A reader and an editor find themselves in the position of having to examine a psychoanalytic paper in terms of a broad range of possibilities, a few salient characteristics of which I have indicated above. I believe that in general the management of a review that serves as the emanation of a scientific society would run its *true risk* if it thought, on the pretext of adopting the theoretical–clinical pluralism currently in vogue, that it had to please everyone, authors and users alike, thus responding to the edifying demands of uniformity and conformity. To push the point: if we did this, we would have a cross between a parish news bulletin and Harlequin's costume. The *most obvious risk*, of course, is that of shoddiness, which would result in a product that would be better off not circulating. The two risks are not mutually exclusive. I do not believe that we have got to this point, but it is worth keeping these risks in mind in our evaluations.

All this is accompanied by a further negative possibility: that for the most varied reasons we lose or blunt our capacity to distinguish between great cuisine and industrial and adulterated foods. "Great cuisine" is as much a rarity in our field as in any other, but the anonymous expert taster and the *Rivista* should at least recognize and encourage well-prepared dishes. Otherwise we would end up putting different "businesses" on the same level, as can be found in certain publications by restaurant owners' associations that simply list all the restaurants in the country without distinction. But the guides that sell well are those that make choices and point out the restaurants that are worth a visit or even a journey. A psychoanalytic review, if it intends to go beyond the restricted function of documenting the scientific activities of its members, must make choices, but it will always be obliged, given the nature of its statutory constraints, to settle for minimal requirements. And yet it can contribute to the improvement of the "business" and the quality of the products offered, from the most humble to the most sophisticated. Its job, then, is to support and guide the author. The task is not an easy one, and it does not fall to the reader alone but to the entire editorial board. I am also convinced that only those who come to terms with the actual work of cooking and with its difficulties will acquire the skills needed for the specific job of analysis and of critical support for the work of other colleagues. The operations involved will always be delicate and to a large extent arbitrary. They require editorial tact and balance, but also the author's willingness to interact with those responsible for the publication. This is where science ends and *taste* begins, though the former can never be reduced to the latter.

I would not like to give the impression in concluding with this gastronomic analogy that I have sought to underestimate the import of the whole problem. Anything but! From the point of view of a connoisseur of fine cuisine and a sometime amateur chef, I have given to the problem the same importance I attribute to the *Rivista*. Our publication must also provide refreshment for the soul. It is not necessary for the entire menu to appeal to everyone, and the customer must be allowed a choice, but there should always be a main dish along with something on the light side and the occasional tasty morsel. As a whole, the dinner should be pleasing and all the courses prepared with care. Otherwise the result will be, if not indigestible, certainly uninteresting; an exclusively documentary function, necessarily marked by little or no selection, will tend to prevail, and we will end up with a dull publication of little interest or appeal to anyone.

NOTES

1. *Entia non sunt multiplicanda praeter necessitatem:* Entities must not be multiplied beyond what is necessary.

CHAPTER SEVEN

The evaluation of psychoanalytical texts and the imaginary scenario in which their writing takes place: observations of an editor

Francesco Barale

Since the editor's point of view is rather different from that of the "readers", I thought I, too, might have a say in the matter of the evaluation of the papers that are sent to the *Rivista*. In the *Rivista*, work is organized in such a way that the first task of the editor, when evaluating an article for publication, is to consider the opinions and comments of the two "readers" of the Board of Readers. These opinions are then reported and compared during the editorial meetings where the editor contributes his own impressions and appraisals.

In this way, the editor works on an "extended" text, composed of the original work under examination, as well as the opinions of those who have read it. The anonymous "readers" (together with the cohort of fantasies as to their identity) assume the role of narrators in this extended text. The editor knows, however, that his general evaluation is just another element contributing to the decision-making procedure; his point of view will be discussed with the second editor also working on the same text, with the entire editorial staff, in the course of regular meetings, and with the chief editor. Issues of political timeliness, which are always detestable and, indeed, detested but, alas, never completely avoidable, may also be taken into consideration.

The editor's function, in this itinerary of readings and evaluations, involves an intricate series of problems (not to mention fantasies, projections, conjectures, competitive opinions, forecasts etc.), on which it could prove interesting to reflect, if one had the time. The fact that the readers' opinions are anonymous gives the editor greater freedom to express his point of view, as it evolves from the readers' opinions via the complex network described above. Not that we must deceive ourselves that this opinion is "objective" or, naively, without prejudice, but at least it is not immediately burdened by institutional issues. When all is over, however, and judgement has been passed, I find it useful and interesting to know who the reader–characters I have worked with in my mind really correspond to, if for no other reason than to see whether I had guessed their identity. But it is not my intention to go into the dynamics of this process in the present chapter.

There is, however, a case that is really very interesting, given the problem we are addressing: that in which the opinions of the two readers concerning the value and/or suitability for publication of the work in question not only fail to coincide but indeed are in direct contrast. This occurrence is not at all rare; in fact, it is rather frequent, if not the norm. It may also happen that the contrast occurs not between the readers' opinions but between the conclusions reached by the two editors separately. The latter may give different interpretations or emphases to the divergences occurring in the readers' evaluations. For the sake of simplicity, let us restrict ourselves to reflecting on the case "diverging opinions of the readers"—surely a worthwhile endeavour. Indeed, this is not such a catastrophic situation, because if, on the one hand, it complicates the editor's task, on the other, it forces him to interact mentally with the conflicting points of view in a far more dynamic way. It prevents him from conforming to the readings already made (as would be easier, following their flow), and forces him to form an idea of his own (or at least a fantasy) concerning the reasons behind the disagreement. Something has obviously happened. To begin with, the minimal criteria for the oft-repeated and apparently fairly simple acceptance of a paper have not been attended to. These concern syntax and grammar, an acceptable logical basis for the views advanced, relevance to psychoanalysis, and a logical conceptual elaboration in full respect of differences of opinions, models, and styles. But these criteria, which are so easy to list, are, in fact, difficult to apply, as anyone with experience of editorial work knows. Indeed, it is enough to consider how many different opinions (which, in turn, involve questions of a more or less epistemological nature, of models, or quite simply of taste) can be expressed among us when we try to establish the necessary characteristics and ingredients within a psychoanalytical text, of acceptable if not convincing argumentation (for example, is purely "narrative" argumentation acceptable?). I am obviously not suggesting we find an impossible common code to eliminate these divergences, which are probably not only unavoidable but perhaps to a certain extent useful. In general, contrasts are useful when they occur in an atmosphere of exchange and reasonable, mutual tolerance. Of course, everyone would appreciate this, but it is seldom achieved. It goes without saying that nobody is the repository of official truth, and in any case the final evaluation of the article usually also benefits from the point of view of the editor (who, however, in the final analysis holds the minority opinion). For example, the author may be asked to modify the text slightly. It is not a question, therefore, of trying to achieve an impossible (and undesirable) homogeneity of evaluations. Rather, by taking all these facts into consideration, it is necessary to reflect on the way in which our evaluations develop and on their foundations.

The case described (contrasting opinions) lends itself, above all, to highlighting the importance of a problem: in the case of a psychoanalytical text, it is particularly difficult to extricate the evaluation concerning the formal correctness and scientific relevance of the "content" from the effect on the reader of other aspects and levels of the text. I am referring to those that exist in every kind of text (e.g. meta-textual, meta-communicative, illocutory, performative, pragmatic–affective, etc.). This can occur simply because the psychoanalyst is highly tuned to these very registers, where what is particularly relevant to psychoanalysis is expressed in its most direct manner. They are true indicators of the imaginary scenario in which writing takes place and of the emotions that play a part in it.

The problem concerns, above all, articles of "average" quality (the majority). In these cases, for example, the effect induced by the above characteristics of the text can be decisive.

I will give an example (radically modified, for reasons of discretion): a work of "average" quality, written in reasonable Italian, sufficiently clear and comprehensible, rich in clinical descriptions, received two contrasting opinions. The first reader, full of praise and favourable to publication, had appreciated its "originality". The second, however, was decidedly negative. Both the editors, despite slight variations, concurred with the latter, and the work was rejected. On a second look at this text and at the appraisals it received, it appears obvious that, in terms of certain aspects (those corresponding to the minimal criteria for publication), the article is really neither better nor worse than many others that are accepted. But I have the impression, on reading it again, that some meta-communicative and meta-textual aspects played an important role in conditioning the different responses (which are directly reflected in the evaluations themselves). The meta-communicative aspect stands out right from the introduction, which sets the tone for all the meta-communication of the work. The introduction is (more or less): "I have decided to call a particular internal organization that I have identified 'hyper Don Giovanni of the Ego ideal', etc. . . ." (Unfortunately, in the necessity to disguise references to the work we lose some of the prosodic effects and the more "heroic *coloritura*" of the original introduction.)

We know that in every text that tells us something, even the most "scientific", most "objective" or apparently most bureaucratic, there is always a meta-communicative aspect involving the author's self-representation and self-promotion.

This can be seen in certain textual devices (and, in the case of more "scientific" texts, paradoxically even in the textual devices that tend to indicate the absolute absence of subjectivity on the part of the narrator towards the "pure facts" narrated). There is a fable (with its relative plot), which is parallel and implicit with the fable (and its plot) of the official content and which, in many ways, consists in variations of a more or less constant nature: given the existence of a problem, or of a set of circumstances to be clarified (that is, an obstacle or a task), the hero—generally, though not necessarily, the narrator—overcomes them in a variety of ways. He shows us how he reaches his goal despite various difficulties, mistakes, uncertainties. If this is true for any text, even the most scientific, it is all the more so in the case of psychoanalytical works, where the narrator's subjectivity is immediately recognized as relevant.

But the ways of implicitly representing (that is, elaborating) this scenario, which runs parallel to the scientific one and which is obviously laden with emotional connotations of immediate psychoanalytical interest (there is Oedipus, of course, along with many other things), are extremely varied. In our case, with his introduction, our author is saying, more or less: "I am comparing myself directly with Freud; I have discovered a series of facts, hitherto unknown, or at least never mentioned before, but which I am now going to take it upon myself to name as a new, original agency. . . ." There is a strong evocation of the virtues and courage of the hero and of his task, which is immediately presented as arduous and original. All would be fine if what follows had not appeared to three readers out of four, perhaps a little irritated by the author's arrogance, as nothing more than a "casual" re-description of internal constellations "regarding which a solid body of psycho-analytical literature exists" as well as an equally well-established terminology (each psychoanalytic school and its variations) with which to describe them. Thus, the Promethean undertaking is brutally inverted into the rather scathing evaluation that the author has simply "discovered hot water".

Yet, I have the impression that the negative opinions the paper in question received were not simply due to the faults officially denounced by the critical readers (lack of originality, little or confused consideration for the literature already in existence concerning the clinical phenomena described, etc.). Seldom does one come across works that are really original, and a casual attitude towards "what has already been written" could also be seen as a quality for the anti-academic spirit it displays. However, it is here, regarding the "tone" of the work, so to speak, that the evaluation, basically of an emotional and psychodynamic nature, is heavily negative. This evaluation obviously springs from the meta-communicative characteristics of the text itself. But I have the impression that even the first reader's positive appraisal is, at least in part, syntonic with a similar order of meta-textual aspects. The implicit declaration of originality of the type: "I use my head when thinking about clinical phenomena and I follow my own ways of thinking, ignoring what has already been said" is reiterated by the author both by means of "original" lexical choices and by the very structure of his arguments. This ignores (in part) the customary models as well as the meta-psychological formulations already in existence and is reflected in the reader's attribution of "originality" (who possibly also approves the implicit choice of a free clinical–theoretical language that invents each time the descriptive categories considered most suitable and evocative).

Another aspect of interest to us is the "constitution of the imaginary reader", as it is called by some students of text analysis. Every text contains its imaginary reader, a figure to whom the author addresses himself and with whom he establishes a relationship (the characteristics of the imaginary reader rarely coincide with those of the actual reader). It is clear that this imaginary interlocutor, who is recognizable in specific textual devices, is of great importance from our point of view. This potential reader (composed largely of the author's projections) is a fundamental part of the writer's imaginary scenario. The style of the author's relationship with this fictitious character (that is, with his own internal imagos) varies within an almost infinite repertoire, as vast as the variety of individual styles.

However, there are some "characters" who may create a problem simply because they conflict with the aversions of the "real" reader (especially if, as in our case, under the obligation imposed by his official position, he cannot escape). Thus, the reader finds himself identified, more or less brusquely, with the imaginary reader. Just to give some personal examples (but the range taken from readers' evaluations could be much wider), I have some difficulties with enigmatic–oracular styles. These are the ones where the author's evaluation is allowed to peep through, here and there, in darting flickers and flashes, in a fleeting and erratic fashion, from sylvan depths of obscurity, like the Being of Heidegger, with the aim of instilling an attitude of ecstatic admiration and idealization (or fierce irritation of a more-or-less envious nature). Worse still, without doubt, are those authors (and they do exist) who establish with their imaginary reader a relationship of the kind "it is the voice of Science that is speaking to you . . ." and the tone becomes stern and lofty . . . the metaphors become heavy-going . . . and the poor reader–psychoanalyst–ignoramus is conceded a few drops of wisdom with a certain, possibly epistemological, condescension. Sometimes difficulties arise from certain seductive–friendly–captivating styles, typical of the "affectionate-good-fellow-no-body-could-say-a-bad-word-about". Worse, though fortunately rare, are certain thundering–hyperbolic styles, as in the case of a colleague, esteemed and liked by all, who once, for some reason, got carried away and sent us some pages in which every second word was written with a capital letter.

I could continue with the anecdotes, and everyone would have his own. From this point of view, one could even attempt a psychoanalytical study of the function of the type of argumentation or even of the figures of classical rhetoric.

But the problem that concerns us directly, in more general terms, is this: the objects of our attention are these texts, these products, and not individuals, who have not asked us for an evaluation. The purpose is to encourage as many colleagues as possible to communicate their thoughts and publish. However, the minimal criteria, to a large extent formal, to which, by explicit agreement, evaluations of texts should adhere, in addition to being far from easy to agree on unanimously, are furthermore constantly contaminated by the effects on the reader induced by other levels of the text: these are laden with emotions and fantasies to which, as analysts, we cannot but attribute great relevance. We may also ask ourselves to what extent this is not legitimate as far as psychoanalytic texts are concerned, where meta-comunicative, pragmatic and emotional aspects (or, more simply, the "tones") are really a very important part of the music.

It is clear that this opens the field to an extreme subjectivity of evaluations and to a confusion or overlapping of levels, and it gives rise to possibly insuperable problems. I am unable to find a clear answer to the question. But I think that a reflection on the mental paths we travel when evaluating could prove useful. It might help us to improve our understanding of the corrections (clearly formal ones) to ask for when necessary. (Obviously, we cannot do analysis or wild semantic analysis of texts and authors, nor can we intervene where personal aspects are concerned; nevertheless, many of the corrections requested are, in fact, often an attempt, conscious or otherwise, to modify meta-communicative or meta-textual aspects.)

I repeat, this problem arises, above all, with papers that, from the formal point of view, would be described as "average" (in the evaluation of which the effect of the above aspects is more important). At the two extremes (excellent work or careless or shoddy work), the problem poses itself differently: I have found myself reluctantly having to propose works for publication that from a formal point of view were faultless and excellently constructed but which I found intolerable for various reasons. On the other hand, unwillingly, I have recommended that works full of stimulating aspects and of the beginnings of original but insufficiently developed thoughts be returned to the author for radical changes.

Finally, I would briefly like to say something about the influence that different theoretical positions and schools of thought have on the evaluations. They are certainly important but, again, heavily conditioned by meta-communicative and meta-textual effects.

Indeed, for the sake of clarity I would say that I have never come across cases in which a below-average work has been praised simply because certain aspects "fall" within fields of particular interest to a reader (or an editor). Conversely, I have never met with cases in which a formally excellent work, with clear objectives, clear arguments, and a clear argumentative structure to sustain them, has received a decidedly negative opinion just because its thesis is in contrast to the theoretical idiosyncrasies of one of the readers. In general, there is tolerance and, at times, genuine curiosity towards different points of view. On the other hand, a critical spirit does not disappear before "family" theses.

Here, too, the problem arises in the case of "average" works. This does not so much concern the opinions expressed or declared (by the author or the reader) but, rather, a level of "secondary importance", so to speak, which once again involves meta-communication and meta-text. Indeed, mainly involved are some of the less evident aspects of the meta-text. Of course, each of us is particularly sensitive to the *shibboleth* he prefers, and perhaps tends to identify it *tout court* with the *shibboleth* of psychoanalysis; but, in fact, we are all aware by now that there are many sub-systems of *shibboleth* that serve to identify different models, theories, groups, and sub-groups . . . And we are well aware, too, that every psychoanalytic text that is sent to us, beknown or not to its author, contains, at one and the same time, a meta-text of *shibboleth*, a set of pointers that serve to indicate implicitly that the author adheres to and shares a particular psychoanalytic sub-language as well as a particular field of thought and so on. [The term *Shibboleth*, a biblical password that permitted recognition not through its content but through the particular accent with which it was pronounced, is used by Freud (in the context of what makes a psychoanalyst immediately recognizable to a non-psychoanalyst) in two passages (1905e [1901], p. 226 fn.;[1] 1911c [1910], p. 7).]

> "And the Gileadites took the passages of Jordan before the Ephraimites: and it was so, that when those Ephraimites which were escaped said, Let me go over; that the men of Gilead said unto him, Art thou an Ephraimite? If he said, Nay; Then said they unto him, say now *Shibboleth* (ear of wheat, or stream): and he said *Sibboleth*: for he could not frame to pronounce it right. Then they took him and slew him at the passages of Jordan" [Judges, 12, 5–6][2]

But this set of pointers, running parallel to the explicit text, is, in turn, composed of various planes. There is a more open and fairly explicit plane (quotations, theoretical references, supported theses, terminological preference, etc.). This level generally creates no problems: we have all become accustomed by now to practising and above all declaring tolerance, with varying degrees of difficulty, of the many psychoanalytic dialects, and we have officially given up hope for a perfect or universal psychoanalytic language. Yet there are other meta-textual planes that function as pointers of "belonging" in a more implicit manner, and these are the ones most often responsible for the differing reactions of the reader. I could quote many examples: the very way in which the author chooses to organize the paper, both formally and in its argumentative structures, may, as I have already mentioned, fulfil this role. This is exemplified by the use of clinical–narrative registers or, vice versa, theoretical–metapsychological registers, or by the various articulations (if present) of these registers . . . and so on, up to the very syntactic and lexical structure. This may apply even more subtly, such as in the use or not of mitigators that may or may not suggest an "unsaturated" discourse or the use of modal pointers that incline one towards a "referential" pole rather than a "constructive-narrative" pole, the "lightness" or "heaviness" of the metaphoric system adopted, the quality and the quantity of explicit presences of the enunciative "I" . . . as well as all the other indicators of *"attachment"* or of the narrator's pre-eminence in describing the "facts" . . . and so on.

Indeed, there are even texts in which meta-communicative and meta-textual aspects predominate to the extent that they seem to represent the real purpose of the paper. In these cases, the text itself is a kind of pretext (forgive the pun) for the meta-communicative and meta-textual aspects. What appears to be of prime importance to the author, in these not at all infrequent cases, is not so much the wish to communicate something he considers new or at least important or to share an experience he has had, as to indicate by means of a series of *shibboleths* that he belongs to a community or a sub-community and wishes to be accepted and recognized as belonging to it by reaffirming its conceptual and linguistic usages and customs and exalting its strengths. In this case, the production of a scientific work tends to resemble its ritual and self-promotional aspects (which, we must remember, are always present to a certain degree). I believe that a great deal of tolerance is due here. Furthermore, as psychoanalysts, we are well aware of the value and function that repetition has in the consolidation of identity.

From this point of view, there are some extremely seductive pieces of writing in which the meta-textual efficacy, in the above-mentioned sense, is at its highest. Yet if, on the one hand, to the reader already familiar with the subject, they may appear wonderful works, to the reader who is uninitiated or even hostile to the system of *shibboleth* itself they can seem intolerable and empty.

Moreover, there is a delicate equilibrium between these different communicative and meta-communicative aspects at various levels of the text. The effect of the particular mixture that each work contains is very subjective. For example, I am irritated both by texts that are excessively saturated by statements in which the author underscores the political line-up to which he belongs, castellated by banners and standards (lexical, syntactic, textual, meta-textual . . .) and by chameleonic texts in which there is an indiscriminate use of different systems of *shibboleth* so as "not to be recognized". Then there are various combinations that sometimes produce jarring effects and where the various meta-textual and meta-communicative levels appear out of tune or even in open discord with one another. Here, again, the repertoire of cases could be lengthy. But I do not want to be long-winded, since my intent was simply to state the problem. There is certainly no need for us to become students of rhetoric or text analysis.

The network of the various levels of phenomena with which a text surrounds us is a complex one. Perhaps it is a good idea to keep this in mind, even if we decide that for our evaluation only one level (perhaps the most superficial) is relevant. In any case, since we are talking of phenomena present to some degree in every text (including this one, of course), my hope is that these reflections give rise to a useful exercise in tolerance.

NOTES

1. The footnote on p. 226 was added in 1920.
2. Although the original German work (*WSF, 11*, 124) contained this passage from the Bible, it does not appear in the *Standard Edition*.

CHAPTER EIGHT

Psychoanalytical visions of reality and styles of writing

Giorgio Sacerdoti

Several years ago, Roy Schafer published an article in the *International Journal of Psycho-Analysis* (1970), subsequently included in his book, "*A New Language for Psychoanalysis*" (1976), in which he outlined four psychoanalytical "visions" of reality described, respectively, as "comic", "romantic", "tragic", and "ironic". If we were simply to ask ourselves to which of these "visions" a large number of the articles written for the *Rivista di Psicoanalisi* in the course of the last ten years might belong (above all, from the stylistic point of view), I believe that, more or less, the romantic vision would have first place. Consequently, it is worth while briefly outlining its main characteristics according to Schafer.

More recently, Strenger (1991) has spoken of the romantic vision in psychoanalysis (to be distinguished from the classical vision) as something that began to develop with Ferenczi. It was taken up again by Balint, developed by Winnicott and, in particular, by Kohut, whose work lends itself excellently to describing the main characteristics of the romantic approach. The tension between "romantic" and "classical" attitudes would seem to reflect a tension that is a fundamental characteristic of human life.

To return to Schafer and to his conceptualization, we are told that life, in the romantic vision, is a quest or a series of quests. The quest is a perilous, heroic, individualistic journey. The destination or goal combines some or all the characteristics of the mystery of the immense, of sacredness, of love and, we could perhaps add, of hatred and possession through—or by fusion with—some higher power or principle.

Supposing that my impression is well-founded and that behind a large proportion of today's psychoanalytical works lies a predominantly "romantic vision", the first thing that occurs to me is to wonder why this should be true right now, and how this fits in with our picture of today's society in general: is it in tune with it or, rather, a "counter-vision in perpetuity", as Erikson (1968) affirms?

Perhaps before attempting to answer this and other questions, it would be wise to illustrate what this impression of a predominantly "romantic" orientation is founded on. To begin with, I would emphasize the fact that in many cases we are dealing with patients who do not fit in with "classical" indications; analysis then appears as an adventurous undertaking that is also more or less heroic. Moreover, the analyst appears to be the epicentre of this undertaking—even if it is part of the bipersonal field. The analyst, in his reports on the progress of the analysis, presents the reader with a picture of what often appears to be disconcertingly heavy, psychosomatic involvement. This is very often related to mechanisms that revolve around projective identification or, sometimes, adhesive identification. If the reader feels inclined to participate in these vicissitudes, one might ask whether sometimes—in addition to the nostalgia for a primitive psychoanalytical heroism—this participation is not perhaps due, in part, to the fear that, by not participating, he might be catalogued as old-fashioned, or, at best, as an old-style Freudian.

In my opinion, it is essential to identify a continuity and a centrality that will allow the majority of readers to recognize in what they read a theoretical–clinical description that is in accordance with an image of psychoanalysis "in progress". This may be easier with styles of writing that avoid unnecessary complications and do not shrink from the facts. The latter are perhaps feared since they risk doing away with the analyst's fantasy. In reference to this, Henry James' "The Real Thing" (1893) excellently renders my point of view. In this novel, a couple of authentic if impoverished members of the upper class visit an artist's studio; after harbouring an initial misapprehension that they had come to order a portrait, the artist accepts them as models since they are just the subjects he has been looking for. Successively he feels his inspiration to be considerably diminished. He opens his eyes to what is happening and dismisses the models only through the intervention of an artist friend who sees the portraits on his return from a journey to a distant country (possibly symbolic of the need for distancing). The protagonist becomes aware of the fact that, with those models, he had too real a picture before his eyes. Consequently he was unable to paint a portrait by drawing on his own phantasy, a painting that could be reinvented by art lovers or by anyone else capable of establishing a link between a personal fantasy (internal reality) and that of others. In this way the protagonist discovers the cruel and perverse law according to which the real thing might be less precious than the imaginary one.

In a certain sense the subjects of James' story are individuals for whom it is true to say, *"le style c'était l'homme"*[1], and who thus leave no room for the style of the artist. The opposite case is that of rather shapeless, presumably structureless, subjects, who ideally leave the sculptor free to follow his own style. The sculptor can, according to Freud, be compared, for certain aspects, with the analyst, in that they both work "*per via di tolle*"[2]. Except, of course, that the analyst does not work on pieces of marble. However, the style, not to mention the content, of many present-day papers (I say many, because " the analyst at work" has become an object-subject increasingly laden with voyeuristic–exhibitionistic aspects) seems, on the whole, so monotonous and repetitive, when not stereotyped, as to render it arduous to believe that these "pieces" are really the fruit of a free encounter and not a superimposition or even imposition. [Rosen (1977) defines "personal style" as being the particular method adopted by an individual in order to use the more or less conventional forms of expression in such a way that the synthesis of the subject (the content) and the form permit the right degree of ambiguity. Thus both subject and object can participate in unravelling the enigma created by this ambiguity.]

After all, we know that the language of an analysis that manages to avoid such snags is peculiar to every analytical couple, despite the fact that the analysing subject remains unchanged. Descriptions of this kind of encounter are not lacking; but I would say that one does not come across them very often when leafing through the *Rivista di Psicoanalisi* of recent years, and the same is true of other journals. They are even absent—though it may seem paradoxical—from the presentations given by candidates applying for membership. In this last case, the kind of writings I mentioned earlier can play an important role, inasmuch as they may heavily influence the candidates. The latter are quick to react with the enthusiasm of the neophyte to what is new or apparently new, scotomizing the fact that sometimes it is really obvious or repetitive.

Risks of the above-mentioned type are reduced in the case of applied psychoanalysis. However, the boundaries between "pure" or theoretical-clinical psychoanalysis and applied psychoanalysis have recently become less clear. This has made a finer definition of the position of the latter essential (a subject dealt with particularly by Tort, 1970, among others). While recognizing that their respective boundaries may be unclear, I think it is important that there should be a constant awareness of which of the two branches we are mainly dealing with.

Finally, the relation between writing and publishing is worth mentioning. A written text may be kept in a drawer (as, for example, Freud's study of transference neuroses)—or it may become the subject of debate in restricted circles, without therefore, becoming formalized in a publication: after all, as we know, *verba volant*![3]

NOTES

1. *Le style c'etait l'homme*: the style was the man.
2. *Per via di tolle:* by carving away.
3. *Verba volant:* the spoken word takes wing.

REFERENCES

Amati-Mehler, J., Argentieri, S., & Canestri, J. (1993). *The Babel of the Unconscious. Mother Tongue and Foreign Languages in the Psychoanalytic Dimension.* Madison, WI: International Universities Press.

Anzieu, D. (1975). *L'auto-analyse de Freud* (2 vols.) Paris: Presses Universitaires de France.

Anzieu, D. (1979). The Sound Image of the Self. *International Revue of Psychoanalysis*, 6: 23–36.

Augustine, St. (1836). *Omnia Opera* (Vols. 2 & 8). Paris: Gaume.

Baron, S., & Pletsch, C. (Eds.) (1985). *Introspection in Biography.* Hillsdale, NJ: The Analytic Press.

Barthes, R. (1964). *Essais critiques.* Paris: Seuil.

Barthes, R. (1975). *Roland Barthes par Roland Barthes.* Paris: Seuil.

Bion, W. R. (1962a). A Theory of Thinking. *International Journal of Psycho-Analysis*, 53 (reprinted in *Second Thoughts.* London: Heinemann, 1967).

Bion, W. R. (1962b). *Learning from Experience.* London: Heinemann.

Cremerius, J. (1979). *Il mestiere dell'analista.* Torino: Boringhieri, 1985.

Eiguer, A. (1993). The Unpredictable. One of the Specific Features of the Analytic Dialogue. *Psychoanalysis in Europe, Bulletin 41*: 17–26.

Erikson, E. H. (1968). *Identity: Youth and Crisis*. London: Faber & Faber.

Elon, A. (1975). *Herzl*. New York: Holt, Rinehart and Winston.

Fenichel, O. (1939). *Problems of Psychoanalytic Technique*. New York: Psychoanalytic Quarterly Inc. Fourth edition, 1941.

Fenichel, O. (1946). *The Psychoanalytic Theory of Neurosis*. London: Routledge and Kegan Paul.

Fink, K. (1993). Distorted Listening and Hearing. *Psychoanalysis in Europe, Bulletin 41*: 7–16.

Freud, S. (1891b). *On Aphasia*. New York: International Universities Press, 1953.

Freud, S. (1895d [1893–95]). *Studies on Hysteria. S.E., 2.*

Freud, S. (1898a). Sexuality in the Aetiology of the Neuroses. *S.E., 3.*

Freud, S. (1900a). *The Interpretation of Dreams. S.E., 4–5.*

Freud, S. (1901a). *On Dreams. S.E., 5.*

Freud, S. (1901b). *The Psychopathology of Everyday Life. S.E., 6.*

Freud, S. (1905c). *Jokes and Their Relation to the Unconscious. S.E., 8.*

Freud, S. (1905d). *Three Essays on Sexuality. S.E., 7.*

Freud, S. (1905e [1901]). Fragment of an Analysis of a Case of Hysteria. *S.E., 7.*

Freud, S. (1910a). Five Lectures on Psycho-Analysis. *S.E., 11.*

Freud, S. (1911c [1910]). Psycho-Analytic Notes on an Autobiographical Account of a Case of Paranoia (Dementia Paranoides). *S.E., 12.*

Freud, S. (1912e). Recommendations to Physicians Practising Psycho-Analysis. *S.E., 12.*

Freud, S. (1914d). On the History of the Psycho-Analytic Movement. *S.E., 14.*

Freud, S. (1915e). The Unconscious. *S.E., 14.*

Freud, S. (1916–17). *Introductory Lectures on Psycho-Analysis. S.E., 15–16.*

Freud, S. (1918b [1914]). From the History of an Infantile Neurosis. *S.E., 17.*

Freud, S. (1920b). *A Note on the Prehistory of the Technique of Analysis. S.E., 18.*

Freud, S. (1920g). *Beyond the Pleasure Principle. S.E., 18.*

Freud, S. (1923b). *The Ego and the Id. S.E., 19.*

Freud, S. (1923c [1922]). Remarks on the Theory and Practice of Dream-Interpretation. *S.E., 19.*

Freud, S. (1925h). Negation. *S.E., 19.*

Freud, S. (1926c). "Foreword" to E. Pickworth Farrow's *A Practical Method of Self-Analysis. S.E., 20.*

Freud, S. (1933a [1932]). *New Introductory Lectures on Psycho-Analysis. S.E., 22.*

Freud, S. (1937c). Analysis Terminable and Interminable. *S.E., 23.*

Freud, S. (1939a). *Moses and Monotheism. S.E., 23.*

Freud, S. (1940a [1938]). *An Outline of Psycho-Analysis. S.E., 23.*

Freud, S. (1941f [1938]). Findings, Ideas, Problems. *S.E., 23.*

Freud, S. (1954). *The Origins of Psychoanalysis.* London: Imago.

Freud, S. (1985). *The Complete Letters of Sigmund Freud to Wilhelm Fliess.* Cambridge. MA: Harvard University Press.

Freud, S., & Jung, C. G. (1974). *Briefwechsel.* Frankfurt/Main: S. Fisher Verlag. [*The Freud/Jung Letters.* William McGuire (Ed.). Princeton, NJ: Princeton University Press, 1974]

Gardner, R. (1983). *Self Inquiry.* Hillsdale, NJ: The Analytic Press, 1989.

Gardner, R. (1994). *On Trying to Teach.* Hillsdale, NJ: The Analytic Press.

Gardner, R. (1995). *Hidden Questions, Clinical Meanings.* Hillsdale, NJ: The Analytic Press.

Gay, P. (1988). *Freud: A Life for Our Time.* New York: Norton.

Gedo, J. (1968). Noch einmal der gelehrte Säugling. *Psyche, 22*: 301–319.

Gedo, J. (1970). Thoughts on Art in the Age of Freud. *Journal of the American Psychoanalytical Association, 18*: 219–245.

Gedo, J. (1972). The Dream of Reason Produces Monsters. *Journal of the American Psychoanalytical Association*, 20: 485–505.

Gedo, J. (1973). Kant's Way. *Psychoanalytic Quarterly, 42*: 409–434.

Gedo, J. (1979). *Beyond Interpretation* (Revised edition). Hillsdale, NJ: The Analytic Press, 1993.

Gedo, J. (1981). *Advances in Clinical Psychoanalysis.* New York: International Universities Press.

Gedo, J. (1983). *Portraits of the Artist* (Paperback edition). Hillsdale, NJ: The Analytic Press, 1989.

Gedo, J. (1984). *Psychoanalysis and Its Discontents.* New York: Guilford.

Gedo, J. (1986). *Conceptual Issues in Psychoanalysis.* Hillsdale: NJ: The Analytic Press.

Gedo, J. (1988). *The Mind in Disorder.* Hillsdale, NJ: The Analytic Press.

Gedo, J. (1991). *The Biology of Clinical Encounters.* Hillsdale, NJ: The Analytic Press.

Gedo, J. (1996). *The Artist and the Emotional World.* New York: Columbia University Press.

Gedo, J., & Gedo, M. (1992). *Perspectives on Creativity.* Norwood, NJ: Ablex.

Gedo, J., & Gehrie, M. (1993). *Impasse and Innovation in Psychoanalysis.* Hillsdale, NJ: The Analytic Press.

Gedo, J., & Goldberg, A. (1973). *Models of the Mind.* Chicago, IL: University of Chicago Press.

Gedo, J., & Pollock, G. (Eds.) (1976). Freud: The Fusion of Science and Humanism. *Psychological Issues, Monograph 34/35.* New York: International Universities Press.

Gedo, M. (1980). *Picasso—Art as Autobiography.* Chicago: University of Chicago Press.

Gedo, M. (1994). *Looking at Art from the Inside Out.* New York & Cambridge: Cambridge University Press.

Gedo, M. (Ed.) (1985). *Psychoanalytic Perspectives on Art,* Vol. I. Hillsdale, NJ: The Analytic Press.

Gedo, M. (Ed.) (1987). *Psychoanalytic Perspectives on Art,* Vol. II. Hillsdale, NJ: The Analytic Press.

Gedo, M. (Ed.) (1988). *Psychoanalytic Perspectives on Art,* Vol. III. Hillsdale, NJ: The Analytic Press.

Grinstein. A. (1980). *Sigmund Freud's Dreams.* New York: International Universities Press.

Haynal, A. (1993). *Psychoanalysis and the Sciences: Epistemology—History.* London: Karnac Books.

Homans, P. (1988). Disappointment and the Ability to Mourn: De-Idealization as a Psychological Theme in Freud's Life, Thought, and Social Circumstances, 1906–1914. In: P. Stepansky (Ed.), *Freud: Appraisals and Reappraisals,* Vol. 2 (pp. 3–101). Hillsdale, NJ: Analytic Press.

Ippolito, G. (1991). Revisione tra pari. Una garanzia di qualità per il giornale scientifico e per il lettore. *Medifax, 1* (1).

James, H. (1893). The Real Thing. In: *The Aspern Papers and Other Stories.* London: Penguin Books, 1976.

Jaques, E. (1981). The Aims of Psychoanalytic Treatment. In: J. S.

Grotstein, *Do I Dare Disturb The Universe*. Beverly Hills, CA: Caesura Press.

Jones, E. (1953–57). *The Life and Work of Sigmund Freud* (Vols. 1–3). New York: Basic Books.

Jones, E. (1959). *Free Associations*. New York: Basic Books.

Lévi-Strauss, C. (1961). *A World on the Wane*. London: Hutchinson.

Lock, S. (1991). Il ruolo della revisione critica nella letteratura biomedica. *Medifax, 1* (I).

Mahony, P. (1979). Friendship and Its Discontents. *Contemporary Psychoanalysis, 15*: 55–109.

Mahony, P. (1982). *Freud as a Writer*. New York: International Universities Press.

Mahony, P. (1984). Further Reflections on Freud and His Writing. *Journal of the American Psychoanalytical Association, 32*: 847–864.

Mahony, P. (1987). *Freud as a Writer* (second enlarged edition). New Haven, CT: Yale University Press.

Mahony, P. (1993). Freud's Cases: Are They Valuable Today? *International Journal of Psycho-Analysis, 74*: 1027–1035.

Masson, J. M. (Ed.) (1985). *The Complete Letters of Sigmund Freud to Wilhelm Fliess, 1887–1904*. Cambridge, MA: The Belknap Press of Harvard University Press.

Moraitis, G., & Pollock, G. (Eds.) (1987). *Psychoanalytic Studies of Biography*. Madison, CT: International Universities Press.

Moscone Ricardo, O. (1993). Indagaciòn al escrito psicoanalitico. *Revista de Psicoanalisis: "Escritura en Psicoanalisis", 49* (1: Jan.–Feb.).

Musatti, C. L. (1976). *Introduzione al Vol. 8 delle Opere di Sigmund Freud*. Torino: Boringhieri.

Olinick, S. L. (1980). *The Psychotherapeutic Instrument*. New York & London: Jason Aronson.

Olinick, S. L. (1982). Meanings beyond Words: Psychoanalytic Perceptions of Silence and Communication. *International Revue of Psychoanalysis, 9*: 461–471.

Olinick, S. L. (1984). Psychoanalysis and Languages. *Journal of the American Psychoanalytical Association, 32*: 617–653.

Ong, W. J. (1982). *Orality and Literacy*. London & New York: Methuen, 1987.

Plato. *The Dialogues of Plato* (transl. B. Jowett). New York: Random House (1892; 1937).

Poland, W. S. (1986). The Analyst's Words. *Psychoanalytic Quarterly, 55*: 244–295.

Reik, T. (1951). *Listening with the Third Ear.* Garden City, NY: Garden City Books.

Rizzuto, A.-M. (1993). Freud's Speech Apparatus and Spontaneous Speech. *International Journal of Psycho-Analysis, 74*: 113–127.

Rosen, V. H. (1977). *Style, Character and Language.* New York: Jason Aronson Inc.

Sandler, J. (1983). Reflections on Some Relations Between Psychoanalytic Concepts and Psychoanalytic Practice. *International Journal of Psycho-Analysis, 64*: 35–45.

Schafer , R. (1970). The Psychoanalytic Vision of Reality. *International Journal of Psycho-Analysis, 51*: 279–297.

Schafer, R. (1976). *A New Language for Psychoanalysis.* New Haven & London: Yale University Press.

Schafer, R. (1983). *The Analytic Attitude.* London: Hogarth Press.

Schafer, R. (1992). *Retelling a Life.* New York: Basic Books.

Spence, D. P. (1982). *Narrative Truth and Historical Truth.* New York & London: W. W. Norton and Co.

Spence, D. P. (1987). *The Freudian Metaphor.* New York & London: W. W. Norton and Co.

Stein, M. H. (1988). Writing about Psychoanalysis, I. *Journal of the American Psychoanalytical Association, 36*: 105–124.

Steiner, G. (1975). *After Babel. Aspects of Language Translation.* Oxford & New York: Oxford University Press (second ed., 1992).

Strenger, C. (1991). *Between Hermeneutics and Science: An Essay on the Epistemology of Psychoanalysis.* Psychological Issues, Monograph 59. International Universities Press.

Tort, M. (1970). La Psychanalyse dans le Materialisme Historique. *Nouvelle Revue de Psychanalyse, 1*: 146–166.

Tuckett, D. (1991). Editorial. *International Journal of Psycho-Analysis, 72*: 377–381.

Tuckett, D. (1994). Some Thoughts on the Presentation and Discussion of the Clinical Material of Psychoanalysis. *International Journal of Psycho-Analysis, 74*: 1175–1189.

Weber, S. (1982). *The Legend of Freud.* Minneapolis, MN: University of Minnesota Press.

Winnicott, D. W. (1958). The Capacity to Be Alone. In: *The Maturational Processes and the Facilitating Environment.* London: Hogarth Press, 1965. [Reprinted London: Karnac Books, 1990.]

INDEX